Fundamentals of Mortality Risks during the Perinatal Period and Infancy

... ~ volumes !

fondly

Svraul

Christmas 1977.

Monographs in Paediatrics

Vol. 9

Series Editors:
F. Falkner, Yellow Springs, Ohio; *N. Kretchmer*, Bethesda, Md.; *E. Rossi*, Bern

Secretaries: *F. Sereni*, Milan; *F. Vassella*, Bern

S. Karger · Basel · München · Paris · London · New York · Sydney

Fundamentals of Mortality Risks during the Perinatal Period and Infancy

Illustrations by a Comparative Study between Göteborg and Palermo

F. Falkner

University of Cincinnati, College of Medicine, The Fels Research Institute,
Yellow Springs, Ohio

In collaboration with:
J. Ashford, Exeter; *J. Fryer*, Exeter; *P. Karlberg*, Göteborg; *A. Priolisi*, Palermo

61 figures and 34 tables, 1977

S. Karger · Basel · München · Paris · London · New York · Sydney

Monographs in Paediatrics

Vol. 6: P.R. Swyer (Toronto, Ont.). With a contribution by M.A. Llewellyn (Toronto, Ont.): The Intensive Care of the Newly Born. Physiological Principles and Practice
X + 208 p., 43 fig., 35 tab., 1975
ISBN 3–8055–2184–7

Vol. 7: R.P. Zurbrügg (Bern): Hypothalamic-Pituitary-Adrenocortical Regulation. A Contribution to Its Assessment, Development and Disorders in Infancy and Childhood with Special Reference to Plasma Cortisol Circadian Rhythm
VIII + 84 p., 49 fig., 14 tab., 1976
ISBN 3–8055–2253–3

Vol. 8: A. Pérez-Soler (Barcelona): The Inflammatory and Atresia-Inducing Disease of the Liver and Bile Ducts
X + 246 p., 17 fig., 11 tab., 1976
ISBN 3–8055–2257–6

Cataloging in Publication
Falkner, Frank
Fundamentals of mortality risks during the perinatal period and infancy: illustrations by a comparative study between Göteborg and Palermo.
F. Falkner, in collaboration with J. Ashford et al. – Basel, New York, Karger, 1977
(Monographs in paediatrics, v.9)
1. Infant, Newborn, Diseases 2. Fetal Death 3. Infant Mortality
I. Ashford, J. II. Title III. Series
W1 MO568G v.9/WS 420 F193f
ISBN 3–8055–2651–2

Contents

Contributors and Collaborators

Prof. *John R. Ashford,* MA, PhD, FBCS, Professor of Statistics and Head, Department of Mathematical Statistics and Operational Research, University of Exeter, Exeter.

Dr. *F.S.W. Brimblecombe,* CBE, FRCP, Consultant Paediatrician, The Royal Devon and Exeter Hospitals, Exeter.

Prof. *Frank Falkner,* MD, FRCP, Fels Professor of Pediatrics, University of Cincinnati College of Medicine; and Director, Fels Research Institute, Yellow Springs, Ohio.

John G. Fryer, BScEcon, PhD, Reader in Statistics, Department of Mathematical Statistics and Operational Research, University of Exeter, Exeter.

Mrs. *J. Finch,* Senior Systems Analyst, Department of Mathematical Statistics and Operational Research, University of Exeter, Exeter.

Philip Fisher, BSc, MSc, (one time) Institute of Biometry, University of Exeter, Exeter.

R.A. Harding, BScEcon, Department of Mathematical Statistics and Operational Research, University of Exeter, Exeter.

Prof. *Petter Karlberg,* MD, Professor of Paediatrics, Department of Paediatrics No. 1, University of Göteborg, Göteborg.

Thorwald Landström, PhD, Computer Systems Consultant, Department of Paediatrics No. 1, University of Göteborg, Göteborg.

Prof. *Antonio Priolisi,* MD, Professor of Child Health, University of Palermo, Palermo.

Urban Selstam, MD, Assistant Professor of Paediatrics, Department of Paediatrics No. 1, University of Göteborg, Göteborg.

Preface

At a conference held under the auspices of the National Institute of Child Health and Human Development concerning Key Issues in Infant Mortality,[1] all participants concluded that there is an urgent need for coordinated studies of infant mortality and morbidity in a wide variety of human populations, using sophisticated epidemiological methods. It was generally agreed that the currently available statistics about infant mortality in different countries are difficult to compare, because of variations in definitions and criteria. A further major obstacle to the assessment of the available data is the lack of information about medical, social and environmental factors which may contribute to infant mortality. Furthermore, reductions in mortality rates which have taken place during recent years have emphasized the positive concept of 'intact survival', as opposed merely to the avoidance of mortality, as the goal of an effective maternity service. At the same time, the general escalation of the costs of providing all forms of medical care has focused attention upon the evaluation of both the inputs of financial and other resources as well as the outputs of the maternity care system. Indeed, a major problem which has emerged is that of selecting the policy for the delivery of maternity and pediatric care which will achieve the best possible levels of outcome in a defined population, for a given level of cost and subject to defined constraints on the availability of resources.

To oversimplify, if you wish to reduce the infant mortality rate in a population, particularly one with limited resources, what are the priorities for concentrating these resources?

Stimulated by these concerns, we planned an investigation with the aim of studying in depth some of the key issues involved. We instituted a study in three European countries and coordinated it from the Fels Division of Pediatric

[1] *Falkner, F.* (ed.): Key issues in infant mortality. Natn. Inst. of Child Health and Human Development (US Government Printing Office, Washington 1970).

Research in the United States. University departments in two cities of comparable size and population, yet with grossly different infant mortality rates, were chosen — Palermo, Sicily, and Göteborg, Sweden. The Department of Mathematical Statistics, University of Exeter, England, had been already engaged on infant mortality surveys in the United Kingdom, and had the responsibility of directing the biometric and epidemiological disciplines involved.

Clearly, launching, coordinating, modifying, analyzing and finally publishing the findings from the study — involving four different countries, the Channel, and the Atlantic — were somewhat hazardous factors. This publication will show how it would not have been possible without a real team spirit and much give-and-take from my collaborators *John Ashford, John Fryer, Petter Karlberg,* and *Antonio Priolisi.* All of us most gratefully received frequent, warm hospitality in the European centers. Dr. *F.S.W. Brimblecombe,* CBE, FRCP, Consultant Paediatrician, The Royal Devon and Exeter Hospitals, graciously acted as Consultant to our project; and a particular organizational burden has fallen on Mrs. *Margaret Humphrey,* Prof. *Ashford*'s secretary, and on Miss *Karen Phelps,* my executive secretary. We are all most grateful.

The Publishers and their staffs have been kind, helpful, and patient to a degree that caused us to hold our breath. The Fels Fund Trustees, who own and operate the Fels Research Institute, were ever generous and encouraging in enabling us to launch the study from the Fels Division of Pediatric Research, University of Cincinnati.

Finally, studies such as these, whatever their final contribution, can lead to admiration of expertise, good biomedical scientific cooperation and firm friendship. I gratefully derived all three.

Yellow Springs, Ohio   *Frank Falkner*

Section I

Monogr. Paediat., vol. 9, pp. 1–23 (Karger, Basel 1977)

Perinatal, Neonatal and Infant Mortality in Two European Cities: An Introduction

J.R. Ashford and F. Falkner

Department of Mathematical Statistics and Operational Research, University of Exeter, Exeter, Devon

I. Introduction

We have been concerned, in addition to areas outlined in the Preface, with the development of a methodology for the analysis of epidemiological data concerning perinatal, neonatal and infant mortality. This paper presents a 'broad-brush' analysis of the results of epidemiological surveys carried out at Göteborg, Sweden, and Palermo, Sicily.

At each city, records were collected of some 12,000–13,000 confinements, using as far as possible standardised techniques for data recording and coding. The reliability of the various items of information has been assessed. As expected, all grades of mortality were substantially higher at Palermo than at Göteborg. The overall rates of late fetal deaths, early neonatal death, perinatal death and late neonatal death were respectively 20, 15, 35 and 12 per 1,000 live and still births at Palermo and 6, 6, 13 and 1 per 1,000 at Göteborg. The corresponding infant mortality rates were 31 and 9 per 1,000 live births. There were substantial variations in mortality rate in terms of place of confinement in Palermo. In particular, amongst the confinements taking place at home and in private nursing homes at Palermo, mortality was only slightly higher than at Göteborg where all confinements took place in one of two hospitals. The variations in mortality in terms of birth weight and multiplicity were assessed and it was found that the greatest relative difference between the two surveys applies to birth weights in the range 3,000–4,500 g, the mortality rates amongst the low weight single and twin births being in closer agreement. The large excess of late neonatal mortality at Palermo appears to be associated with infectious diseases, which have no significant effect at Göteborg. The presentation and interpretation of the results will be carried out in the context of the effects of birth weight and multiplicity and recommendations are made concerning an appropriate structure for the comparison of neonatal epidemiological studies in different populations.

The comparison of vital statistics from different countries has a long history and there is no doubt that the results of such studies have been generally useful. Not only do international comparisons permit extrapolation beyond the limits of the situation within any particular country, but also they provide some guidance about which particular features of health care are likely to be important on the basis of generalisation from the existing variety of systems. There are, however, many factors which must be taken into account before the assumption can be made that figures derived from different administrative systems and covering different medical and socio-economic backgrounds are in fact comparable. In the field of perinatal and neonatal mortality, the effects of differences in definitions and conventions of recording are well-known. Although agencies such as the World Health Organisation have made great efforts to standardise the procedures used in the collection and presentation of vital statistics, much still remains to be done before the 'league tables' showing the relative positions of different countries in respect of factors such as perinatal mortality can be taken at face value. Furthermore, in tabulations of data derived from birth and death registration systems in different countries, it may not be possible to cover all aspects of the situation which are likely to be important.

In an attempt to overcome some of these difficulties, detailed, coordinated epidemiological studies have been made of infant mortality in two European cities — Göteborg in Sweden and Palermo in Sicily, with particular emphasis upon perinatal and neonatal mortality. These particular cities are comparable in size, but exhibit substantial differences in socio-economic and environmental factors, in the delivery of medical care and in overall mortality rates. The programme has been carried out by university departments in the two cities and the University of Exeter, England has been responsible for the statistical analysis. The Fels Research Institute's Division of Paediatric Research, University of Cincinnati, has planned and supported the project to date. The specific and primary aims of the study are to identify and assess the levels of perinatal and neonatal mortality in terms of the associated factors, with particular reference to maturity (and its determinants) and other biological, environmental and medical influences. In this way, it is hoped that the results may be capable of generalisation to the situation in the United States and elsewhere. The present paper is concerned with a general description of the survey methods and the main findings of these surveys. More detailed analyses of specific topics will be reported in this monograph and elsewhere.

II. Survey Methods

Biometric Issues

The programme of research consists essentially of field studies of defined populations in Göteborg and Palermo. Although because of variations in local circumstances the two studies differ in design, the same general principles and the same definitions and standards apply. In either case, the population under investigation consists of all births taking place to mothers normally resident in particular geographical areas. For each such birth, information is recorded concerning the characteristics of the mother, the mother's previous pregnancies, the present pregnancy, the delivery and the new-born infant. In Palermo, this information was collected by a team of field workers specially recruited for the purpose. The corresponding information for the Göteborg survey was obtained from a standard obstetric and child health record maintained for each pregnancy by the staff of the local health care system. The items of information collected on the two surveys are summarised in appendix 1.

Göteborg Survey

Göteborg is the second largest city in Sweden with a population of about 460,000. There are approximately 6,000 births per annum and virtually all mothers are delivered in hospital. There are two maternity hospitals — the East and West Hospitals — and one children's hospital. Until January 1973, the children's hospital was situated in close proximity to the West Hospital: this unit was replaced by a new children's hospital situated in proximity to the East Hospital. Each of the maternity hospitals includes a neonatal unit with 20 beds, and some new-born infants are referred to the infant ward or to the intensive care ward at the Children's Hospital. The Maternity and Child Welfare Service is all-embracing and is provided free of charge. During a normal pregnancy, three or four ante-natal examinations by an obstetrician are the general rule but, if necessary, further examinations are made. A post-partum follow-up takes place 6–8 weeks after delivery and further consultations are arranged if complications arise. The expectant mother is also under the care of a midwife throughout the whole of the pregnancy and post-partum period.

The information available is based upon a medical birth record developed at the West Hospital. In 1972, this record was accepted by the Swedish Health Board as the first part of a new standard individual record. From January 1973, these records have been used for the clinical management of the mother and child, and are completed for all mothers delivered in all maternity hospitals in Sweden. The present paper is concerned with the results obtained at the West and East Hospitals during the 2-year period 1972–73. At the East Hospital, the standard record for 1972 was constructed retrospectively from the current hospital records, which proved adequate for the purpose.

Table I. Population survey in terms of place of delivery and numbers of births

(a) Göteborg (1972–73)

Place of delivery	Number	%
West Hospital	5,585	45.5
East Hospital	6,686	54.5
Total	12,271	100

(b) Palermo (November 1971 to October 1972)

Place of delivery	Type of record								Total	
	Standard		University Hospital		Public Hospital		Statistics Office			
	number	%	number	%	number	%	number	%	number	%
University Hospital	557	4.2	521	4.0	–	–	21	0.2	1,099	8.3
Public Hospital A	622	4.7	–	–	649	4.9	437	3.3	1,708	13.0
Public Hospital B	881	6.7	–	–	472	3.6	33	0.2	1,386	10.5
Public Hospital A or B	0	0.0	–	–	–	–	634	4.8	634	4.8
Private clinic	2,612	19.8	–	–	–	–	2,382	18.1	4,994	37.9
Home	1,052	8.0	–	–	–	–	2,180	16.5	3,232	24.5
Unknown	10	0.1	–	–	–	–	125	0.9	135	1.0
Total	5,734	43.5	521	4.0	1,121	8.5	5,812	44.1	13,188	100.0

The survey population is defined in terms of mothers normally resident within the geographical area covered by the City of Göteborg and delivered at either hospital during the relevant period. Most mothers are discharged from hospital within 10 days of admission and the information about neonatal and infant mortality was supplemented by reference to the local birth and death registration systems. Virtually all mothers normally living in Göteborg are delivered at one or other of the two hospitals and the survey results apply effectively to the whole population. The various items of information from Göteborg (as summarised in appendix 1) play an integral part in the provision of clinical care for the mother and infant. The accuracy of the individual observations has been found to be high and incomplete records occur only rarely. The survey population is summarised in table I, which shows that about half the births took place at each hospital during the 2-year period.

Deaths taking place to infants after the mother was discharged from hospital would not necessarily be recorded on the hospital record, but details were obtained from the Swedish death registration system. This procedure covers only the deaths which took place (and were registered) in Göteborg, but it is believed that virtually all such deaths to the survey population were included.

Palermo Survey

Palermo is the largest city in Sicily, with a population of about 650,000 and about 13,000 births per year. There is no comprehensive system of maternity care and standards are very variable. Mothers may be delivered in hospital, in private maternity clinics or at home, the choice of place of confinement being determined largely by the patient's ability to pay, by availability of service and the intangible personal preference and attitude of the mother. There are three maternity hospitals, of which one is the University Hospital and the remainder are public hospitals. The public and university hospitals work under very severe pressure of demand and the facilities provided at the University Hospital are probably superior. There are 13 private maternity clinics, which provide very variable standards of care. There are no ante-natal clinics in the sense they are known in the United States, Sweden or England. Each of the districts into which the municipality of Palermo is divided has the services of a general practitioner (medico condotto) and one or more domiciliary midwives.[1]

Infants of low birth weight or new-born babies in distress are sent to the Children's Hospital neonatal section, or to the neonatal section of the Child Health Institute. There is no neonatal resuscitation unit. Comparative and standardised maternity records do not exist, and the Palermo survey is based upon a systematic enquiry by staff specially recruited for the purpose.

[1] These services in fact are available for the unemployed and designated 'poor'. For those who are employed, medical services are available and obtained from personnel listed in one of the several appropriate national and local health schemes.

The population under study at Palermo comprises mothers normally resident in the Administrative Area of Palermo, which is divided into 21 districts. The majority of the births in this population are registered at the Main Registration Office, but there are also 13 peripheral registration offices. The choice of a particular registration office is at the discretion of the person registering the birth and is normally made on the basis of ease of access. All still births, neonatal and infant deaths are registered at the Main Registration Office. By law, births must be registered within 10 days after delivery. Still births, neonatal and infant deaths must be registered within 24 h.

It was originally intended to cover the whole population of births, but experience soon showed that this was not possible with the limited resources available. In the event, the choice of subjects for assessment on the survey was conditioned by two main factors – ease of contact and the need to obtain a comprehensive cover of all places of delivery. At the University Hospital and the two public hospitals, it was intended that all the mothers should be included, up to a limit of ten per day at each hospital. All the mothers delivered at the private clinics were also to be covered and, in either case, the mother's area of normal residence was recorded. As far as the domiciliary confinements are concerned, all mothers whose delivery was registered at either the Main Registration Office or at either of two selected peripheral registration offices were visited by the survey team. All still births and neonatal deaths to mothers normally resident in the Administrative Area were subject to a special enquiry, lists of the mothers concerned being obtained from the Main Registration Office.

Details of death of infants occurring between the 29th day and the first year of life were also obtained from the Main Registration Office and were linked to the corresponding information about the birth. It is possible that some children born in Palermo may have left the city subsequently and may have died before reaching one year of age. In this case, the death would not be registered at Palermo, but if the death took place in Italy, information would be returned to the Palermo Registration Office. However, the number of deaths which would not be reported under this system is believed to be negligible.

Following a short pilot study, the survey proper began in November 1971 and continued for one calendar year, apart from a break during the month of August 1972 for staff holidays. During this month, data were obtained retrospectively from records (appendix 1). The cover achieved is summarised in terms of place of confinement in table I. Out of about 13,000 births taking place during the survey year, just under half were covered by the detailed survey enquiry and so-called 'standard' records were completed. Less complete information was collected for the remainder of the deliveries on a retrospective basis, the sources of information being the hospital record or (for births which did not take place in hospital) the birth registration particulars. This process has resulted in three further types of record – University Hospital, Public Hospital and

Statistics Office — which include progressively less detailed information, as indicated in appendix 1. Reference to table I shows that for some 634 births registered as having taken place in a public hospital, the appropriate hospital records were not located. It is not therefore possible to assign the corresponding records to one or other of the two public hospitals and the group has been considered separately. In total, about 44% of deliveries were covered by each of the Standard and Statistics Office records, 8% by Public Hospital records and 4% by University Hospital records. In terms of place of confinement, some 38% of births took place in a private clinic, 25% at home, 29% at one or other of the public hospitals and the remaining 8% at the University Hospital.

Thus, the most detailed and specific information was obtained for less than half the total number of births. There are three main reasons for failure to include particular births: (1) deliberate exclusion as part of the data collection programme (e.g. deliveries registered at 11 of the 13 peripheral registration offices); (2) refusal on the part of the mother and/or her medical attendant to participate in the study, or (3) failure on the part of the survey team to make contact with the mother due, for example, to pressure of work or to staff holidays. On general grounds, it can be asserted that the choice of place of delivery reflects particular attributes of the mother and her family. By the same token, it is reasonable to assert that the mothers who refused to take part in the survey are likely to differ in certain respects from the remainder of the population. Comparisons of the distribution of items of information common to all four types of record confirm that there are in fact significant differences between the samples covered by each type. When items which are not covered on each type of record are considered, it is necessary to apply appropriate corrections on a statistical basis in order to obtain results which can be applied with confidence to the whole population (appendix 2). However, the analyses described in the present paper refer only to items common to all types of record and this reservation does not apply. It is, however, clear that because of differences in the basic sources of data, the accuracy of any particular item may vary from one type of record to another.

For all deliveries in hospital resulting in a live birth which were covered by the Standard Records, the mother concerned was interviewed by a hospital midwife and a standard series of questions was put to her. A similar form of enquiry was used for deliveries taking place in the private clinics or at home, the mother being visited by a medical social worker as soon as practicable after the birth and almost invariably within 3 weeks. In the case of still births and neonatal deaths, the mother was interviewed by a medically qualified Research Fellow and the standard enquiry, together with a further series of questions about the infant death, was carried out. Due to the virtual absence in Palermo of post-mortem examinations, the cause of death listed is a clinical diagnosis. In order to identify each case and to provide control over the conduct of the survey, a special survey registration number was allocated sequentially to each birth registered to mothers normally resident in the Administrative Area, a specially trained secretary visiting each appropriate Registration Office on alternate days.

The content of the standardised enquiry is summarised in appendix 1. Information was recorded concerning the mother, her past obstetric history, the current pregnancy, the delivery, the infant and the father. For still births and neonatal deaths, the cause of death (as far as this was possible) and other factors concerning the delivery and the circumstances of the death were ascertained. In view of the wide range of conditions experienced before and during the pregnancy, delivery and neonatal periods, a detailed record was made of the past obstetric history and of the employment and smoking habits of the mother during the pregnancy, of the care received before, during and after the delivery. In order to provide a general indication of the environment and life-style experienced by the mother since her own childhood, the occupation and employment of the child's father was recorded, in addition to appropriate data on the mother (appendix 1). Data on the father was subsequently coded and assessed in terms of the classification of occupation and social status used in the United Kingdom.

Infants delivered in hospital are normally weighed at birth, but this information may not be recorded for domiciliary confinements. During the visit to the mother following a delivery at home or in a private clinic, the medical social workers were therefore required to record the weight of the infant, using portable balances which were regularly checked and standardised. For births taking place in each hospital, the same portable balances were used to weigh infants.

The Palermo survey has been carried out by a team of three doctors, two hospital midwives, four medical social workers and one secretary. Great care has been taken to ensure the comparability and (where possible) the validity of all the items of information collected, by means of preliminary training programmes, pilot trials and regular checks upon individual performance.

III. Outcome of Delivery

In the analysis of the results of the survey, we have considered the following indicators of mortality: (a) late fetal death — at least 28 weeks of gestation and no evidence of life at birth; (b) early neonatal death — live-born, but dead within the first 7 days of life; (c) perinatal death — the sum of a and b above; (d) late neonatal death — live-born, but dead between 7 and 28 days of life; (e) neonatal death — the sum of b and d above; (f) death following live birth between 28 days and one year of life, and (g) infant mortality — the sum of e and f above.

The mortality rates for items a to d have been calculated on the basis of the total number of late fetal deaths and live births. On the other hand, the rates e to g have been calculated on the basis of the number of live births, late fetal

Table II. Outcome of pregnancy in terms of place of delivery: rate per 1,000 births (rounded figures)

Place of delivery	Late fetal death (1)	Early neonatal death (1)	Perinatal death (1)	Late neonatal death (1)	Neonatal death (2)	Deaths between 1 month and 1 year (2)	Infant deaths (2)
Göteborg							
West Hospital	9	6	15	1	7	1	8
East Hospital	5	7	11	0	7	3	10
Both	6	6	13	1	7	2	9
Palermo							
University Hospital	29	21	50	13	35	1	36
Public Hospital A	49	35	83	29	67	7	74
Public Hospital B	32	25	56	18	44	4	48
Public Hospital A or B	46	9	55	3	13	0	13
Private clinic	8	7	15	6	14	2	16
Home	11	7	18	7	14	5	19
All	20	15	35	12	27	4	31

(1) = Rate per 1,000 live and still births; (2) = rate per 1,000 live births.

deaths being excluded. In the commentary on the results, the differences within the two populations to which attention is drawn are in general significant at the 1% level at least. Special mention is made of differences associated with lower levels of significance where appropriate.

The mortality rates observed on the two surveys are summarised in terms of place of delivery in table II. The main feature of these results is the gross difference in all grades of mortality between the two cities. The perinatal mortality rate at Palermo is almost three times as high as at Göteborg, whereas the late neonatal mortality rate is more than ten times as high. On the other hand, mortality between one month and one year is less than twice as high at Palermo.

Within the two cities, there are marked variations in mortality between the different places of confinement. The late fetal death rate at the West Hospital at Göteborg is almost twice as high as at the East Hospital, the difference being significant at the 1% level. However, the early neonatal death rates are in close agreement and when perinatal mortality is considered, the difference between the two hospitals just fails to attain the conventional level of statistical significance (p = 0.10). The late neonatal mortality rates are uniformly low, but the death rate between one month and one year is significantly higher (p = 0.01) for deliveries at the East Hospital. In contrast, the infant mortality rates at the two hospitals do not differ significantly.

At Palermo, all the mortality rates show very substantial variations between the different places of confinement. For births taking place at the private clinics and at home, the levels of perinatal death are very similar to those prevailing at Göteborg. However, the late neonatal mortality amongst these two groups is six times as great as at Göteborg. In contrast, the mortality amongst hospital births is very considerably higher than at Göteborg and the results for Public Hospital A are consistently worse than for the University Hospital or for Public Hospital B. The range of perinatal mortality rates is indeed very wide, from 15 to 83 per 1,000 live and still births. The results for confinements taking place at one or other of the public hospitals (the precise location being unknown) suggest that the lack of information about which of the two hospitals was involved may be associated with the outcome of delivery. However, the numbers concerned are too small to invalidate the figures for the two hospitals separately and there is no doubt that there are real and substantial differences between them. The late neonatal mortality rates show a positive association with perinatal mortality, with the highest figure of 29 per 1,000 live and still births at Public Hospital A.

IV. Birth Weight and Outcome of Delivery

Mortality rates show wide variations both within and between the two populations. It is well-known that within a population, maturity and mortality are closely associated and that the most reliable single indicator of maturity available from data of this type is birth weight. Birth weight was recorded for virtually all births on both surveys and the relation between perinatal mortality and birth weight is summarised in table III, which is sub-divided in terms of single births and twins.

Reference to table III a shows that the majority of the single births weighed between 3,000 and 4,000 g, the proportion decreasing with increasing distance from the central part of the distribution. For the most part, the recorded mortality rates show a general tendency to decrease with increasing birth weight up to 4,500 g and to increase in the two highest birth weight groups. The variation with birth weight is very marked. For example, at Göteborg, perinatal mortality falls from 818 per 1,000 live and still births in the under 1,000 g group to below 1 per 1,000 for birth weights of between 4,501 and 5,000 g. Infant mortality rates at Göteborg show a similar variation. When the perinatal mortality rates in the two cities are compared, it is interesting that the levels for the under 1,500 g birth weight groups are in close agreement. However, as the birth weight increases, the mortality rate at Palermo is an increasing multiple of that at Göteborg, so much so that for birth weights of between 3,001 and 5,000 g the ratio is of the order of 5 to 1. In contrast, perinatal mortality for the highest (over 5,000 g) birth weights is almost three times as high as Göteborg, although because of the small numbers involved (particularly at Göteborg) too much reliance should not be placed upon this result. Late neonatal mortality rates for birth weights above 2,000 g at Palermo also show a tendency to decrease with increasing birth weight, whilst at Göteborg the numbers of deaths are so low that no persistent trend is apparent. For birth weights below 2,000 g, the late neonatal mortality rates on both surveys are effectively constant. Possibly this is a reflection of the fact that the less viable infants in this range of birth weights will have died before reaching the age of 7 days. Mortality between one month and one year shows only a weak association with birth weight, possibly for the same reason. For birth weights of between 3,000 and 4,000 g, mortality between one month and one year is more than twice as high at Palermo than at Göteborg.

Table III b shows the birth weight-mortality relation for twins, of which there were 116 pairs at Göteborg and 133 pairs at Palermo. In each city, the proportion of twin births was about 1 in 50, so that the numbers of cases involved in the calculation of the mortality rates in the various birth weight groups are small and the results should therefore be treated with reserve. There was one set of triplets at Göteborg and four sets of triplets at Palermo. In both cities, the majority of twins weigh between 2,000 and 3,500 g, in contrast to the single births who are on average substantially heavier. There is a general tendency for late fetal, early neonatal and perinatal mortality rates to decrease with increasing birth weight. In general, the perinatal mortality rates for Palermo are very much higher than at Göteborg. Comparison of the bottom rows of

Table III. Outcome of pregnancy in terms of birth weight: rate per 1,000 births

Birth weight g	Number of births		Late fetal death (1)		Early neonatal death (1)		Perinatal death (1)		Late neonatal death (1)		Neonatal death (2)		Death between 1 month and 1 year (2)		Infant death (2)	
	Göt.	Pal.	Göt.	Pal.	Göt.	Pal.	Göt.	Pal.	Göt.	Pal.	Göt.	Pal.	Göt.	Pal.	Göt.	Pal.
(a) Single births																
Under 1,001	33	39	303	231	515	538	818	769	0	26	750	733	42	0	792	733
1,001–1,500	45	65	244	308	333	308	578	615	44	185	452	711	32	0	484	711
1,501–2,000	101	119	79	176	89	160	168	336	39	193	140	429	0	0	140	429
2,001–2,500	326	339	37	47	15	62	52	109	0	68	16	136	6	6	22	142
2,501–3,000	1,631	1,503	6	25	6	10	12	35	0	15	6	25	3	4	9	29
3,001–3,500	4,307	4,213	2	14	1	5	3	20	0	5	1	11	2	4	3	15
3,501–4,000	3,978	4,177	2	10	1	4	3	13	0	3	1	6	2	4	3	10
4,001–4,500	1,357	1,316	1	12	1	6	3	18	0	2	1	8	1	0	3	8
4,501–5,000	278	420	0	19	0	5	0	24	0	2	0	7	0	2	0	10
5,001 and over	13	97	154	41	0	10	154	52	0	10	0	22	0	0	0	22
Unknown	0	622	–	38	–	45	–	84	–	13	–	60	–	8	–	69
Total	12,039	12,910	6	20	5	13	11	33	0	10	6	24	2	4	8	27

Table III (continued)

Birth weight g	Number of births		Late fetal death (1)		Early neonatal death (1)		Perinatal death (1)		Late neonatal death (1)		Neonatal death (2)		Death between 1 month and 1 year (2)		Infant death (2)	
	Göt.	Pal.	Göt.	Pal.	Göt.	Pal.	Göt.	Pal.	Göt.	Pal.	Göt.	Pal.	Göt.	Pal.	Göt.	Pal.
(b) Twins																
Under 1,001	7	5	143	200	857	800	1,000	1,000	0	0	1,000	1,000	0	0	1,000	1,000
1,001–1,500	14	13	214	0	286	462	500	462	0	385	363	846	0	0	363	846
1,501–2,000	21	47	48	43	48	128	96	170	0	298	50	444	0	0	50	444
2,001–2,500	55	65	18	15	18	0	36	15	0	62	19	62	0	0	19	62
2,501–3,000	69	68	14	29	0	29	14	59	0	29	0	61	0	0	0	61
3,001–3,500	55	37	18	54	0	27	18	81	0	29	0	29	0	0	0	29
3,501–4,000	9	11	0	0	0	0	0	0	0	0	0	0	0	0	0	0
4,001–4,500	0	2	–	0	–	0	–	0	–	0	–	0	–	0	–	0
4,501–5,000	2	1	0	0	0	0	0	0	0	0	0	0	0	0	0	0
5,001 and over	0	0	–	–	–	–	–	–	–	–	–	–	–	–	–	–
Unknown	0	17	–	176	–	176	–	353	–	59	–	286	–	0	–	286
Total	232	266	34	41	52	83	86	124	0	98	54	188	0	0	54	188

(1) = Rate per 1,000 live and still births; (2) = rate per 1,000 live births.

Table IV. Perinatal mortality in terms of place of delivery and birth weight: rate per 1,000 live and still births

Place of delivery	Single births: birth weight, g											Twins: all birth-weights
	under 1,001	1,001– 1,500	1,501– 2,000	2,001– 2,500	2,501– 3,000	3,001– 3,500	3,501– 4,000	4,001– 4,500	4,501– 5,000	5,001 and over	all	
Göteborg												
West Hospital	944	571	118	75	12	3	3	2	0	250	13	130
East Hospital	667	583	220	30	12	4	2	4	0	0	10	57
Palermo												
University Hospital	857	583	400	143	54	25	19	47	53	0	46	167
Public Hospital A	818	708	351	139	78	45	39	43	32	0	78	214
Public Hospital B	818	500	474	137	33	32	21	50	0	182	50	190
Public Hospital A or B	666	1,000	750	0	97	42	19	17	87	333	53	200
Private clinic	750	444	214	101	12	10	6	7	24	48	14	71
Home	333	600	280	72	13	10	11	13	13	0	18	0

table IIIa and b shows that overall mortality rates are substantially higher amongst the twins than the single births. However, for birth weights of between 1,500 and 2,500 g, the twins have the better survival record. It is interesting that there were no late neonatal deaths amongst twins at Göteborg, whereas the corresponding rate for Palermo was approximately 100 per 1,000 live and still births when all birth weights are taken together.

V. Place of Confinement, Birth Weight and Outcome of Delivery

We have shown that mortality rates in the two cities vary between different places of delivery. In order to explore these differences in more detail, perinatal mortality rates have been calculated in terms of birth weight and place of delivery as indicated in table IV, which is sub-divided in terms of single births and twins and (for single births only) in terms of birth weight. At Göteborg there is no consistent difference between the two hospitals for single births, although the perinatal mortality for twins was twice as high at the West Hospital than at the East Hospital. At Palermo, on the other hand, mortality amongst births taking place at home and in private clinics is consistently lower than that amongst hospitals births. When the hospitals are compared, the results for Public Hospital A are not consistently different from those for the other hospitals for birth weights of below 2,500 g or above 4,000 g. However, perinatal mortality at this hospital is substantially higher in the range 2,500–3,999 g, which covers the majority of births. The results for twins reflect those for single births very closely, although the overall mortality levels tend to be substantially higher. It is interesting that all 34 twins born at home survived to reach one year of age.

On the basis of these results, it is clear that the differences in overall perinatal mortality rates between the different places of birth persist to a considerable extent when the data are sub-divided in terms of multiplicity and birth weight. However, because of the marked variation of mortality with birth weight, part of the differences in overall mortality may be due to differences in the distributions of birth weight. Thus, populations with a relatively high proportion of low weight births will, all other things being equal, tend to exhibit a higher overall level of mortality than populations with a lower proportion. The distribution of birth weight in terms of place of delivery is summarised in table Va and b which refer respectively to single and twin births. When the two surveys are compared, the birth weight distributions for single births are in close agreement thoughout almost the whole of the range. Some 42 per 1,000 live and still birth weights were below 2,501 g at Göteborg and 46 per 1,000 at Palermo. The proportion of births weighing more than 4,500 g was 22 per 1,000 at Göteborg and 42 per 1,000 at Palermo. The birth weight distributions for the two hospitals at Göteborg are very similar. On the other hand, there are wide variations at Palermo.

Table V. Birth weight in terms of place of delivery: rate per 1,000 live and still births

Place of delivery	Birth weight, g									
	under 1,001	1,001– 1,500	1,501– 2,000	2,001– 2,500	2,501– 3,000	3,001– 3,500	3,501– 4,000	4,001– 4,500	4,501– 5,000	5,001 and over
(a) Single births										
Göteborg										
West Hospital	3	4	9	29	140	358	324	110	22	1
East Hospital	2	4	8	25	132	357	336	115	20	1
Both	3	4	8	27	135	358	330	113	21	1
Palermo										
University Hospital	7	12	5	35	166	394	270	86	19	5
Public Hospital A	7	16	25	49	174	366	260	79	21	2
Public Hospital B	9	6	15	41	170	345	309	79	18	9
Public Hospital A or B	5	3	6	21	100	382	340	97	37	10
Private clinic	1	2	6	21	102	342	367	120	35	4
Home	1	3	8	22	100	308	371	122	50	16
All	3	5	10	28	122	343	340	107	34	8

Table V (continued)

Place of delivery	Birth weight, g									
	under 1,001	1,001– 1,500	1,501– 2,000	2,001– 2,500	2,501– 3,000	3,001– 3,500	3,501– 4,000	4,001– 4,500	4,501– 5,000	5,001 and over
(b) Twins										
Göteborg										
West Hospital	22	65	87	217	359	196	43	0	11	0
East Hospital	36	57	93	250	257	264	36	0	7	0
Both	30	60	91	237	297	237	39	0	9	0
Palermo										
University Hospital	0	86	143	286	257	200	29	0	0	0
Public Hospital A	29	143	229	257	171	86	57	0	29	0
Public Hospital B	51	51	333	128	205	179	0	51	0	0
Public Hospital A or B	0	0	0	556	222	222	0	0	0	0
Private clinic	21	21	144	330	278	144	62	0	0	0
Home	0	0	161	129	516	129	65	0	0	0
All	20	52	189	261	273	148	44	8	4	0

The proportions of low weight (less than 2,500 g) births were 97 per 1,000 at Public Hospital A, 71 per 1,000 at Public Hospital B, 59 per 1,000 at the University Hospital, 34 per 1,000 for home births and 30 per 1,000 for births at private clinics. The home births and births in private clinics show a considerable excess of infants weighing 4,000 g or more. The birth weight distribution of twins shows marked variation between the two cities, the proportion of births weighing less than 2,501 g being 418 per 1,000 at Göteborg and 522 per 1,000 at Palermo. There are also variations between different places of confinement. In particular, at Palermo only 290 per 1,000 of the twins born at home weighed less than 2,500 g.

VI. Cause of Death

Each late fetal death or death following live birth in the two cities was classified in terms of cause of death. Whilst the quality of the resulting information is likely to vary between the two cities and between the various types of record at Palermo, the results give a useful if crude indication of the frequency of occurrence of the main factors associated with mortality. On both surveys, asphyxia after birth was a major cause of early neonatal death, together with respiratory distress at Palermo and the hyaline membrane syndrome at Göteborg, but these two latter causes may in fact overlap to some extent. More than half of the late neonatal deaths at Palermo were attributed to enteritis, sepsis or broncho-pneumonia, whereas these causes are not significant at Göteborg. The diagnosis of broncho-pneumonia also applied to almost half the deaths between one month and one year at Palermo. On this basis, the spectrum of causes of death differs very markedly between the two surveys. At least part of the excess of late neonatal deaths at Palermo can be attributed to infections, which are apparently not a problem in this respect at Göteborg.

VII. Comment

The results described in this paper represent merely a preliminary study of the information collected on the two surveys. They do, however, serve to illustrate certain important points concerning the reliability of the data and the way in which the results of epidemiological surveys of the outcome of delivery in human populations should be analysed and presented (appendix 2).

In the first place, it is necessary to define the population under consideration. We have decided to reject all fetal deaths not reaching a gestational age of 28 completed weeks or more before delivery, by all mothers normally resident in two geographical areas. For the majority of births there is little doubt that the

28-week qualifying gestational age has been attained. For some low weight or immature births, however, there may be real uncertainty about the precise date of conception and the decision as to whether or not a particular birth should be included may depend both upon the mother's recollection and upon the assumptions used to calculate the date of conception. The criteria applied may vary with the characteristics of the mother and her medical attendant.

A second complication is introduced by the use of a classification of mortality which distinguishes between still births and death following live birth. The importance of applying precise criteria in this context is well-known and the definitions recommended by WHO give considerable emphasis to this point. However, a precise definition on paper does not necessarily guarantee uniformity of application by different medical attendants in circumstances in which the financial and other implications to the mother and her family may be affected by whether or not the birth is classified as an abortion, a late fetal death or a death following live birth.

Both potential sources of error may affect the numbers of late fetal deaths and early neonatal deaths recorded on the surveys. The ratio of these two quantities is a useful indicator of possible discrepancies in this respect. This ratio is 1.5 at the West Hospital at Göteborg, in contrast to 0.71 at the East Hospital. The two hospitals are separated by a distance of less than five miles and both are well-staffed and well-equipped, with a mortality record which is low by any standards. The catchment areas of the two hospitals are very similar in terms of socio-economic conditions and it is thought that the most likely explanation of this discrepancy is that different conventions have been applied. In view of the very small numbers of infants born at about 28 weeks of gestation, inaccuracies in the calculation of gestational age are probably less important than the application of inconsistent standards for the assessment of live birth at the two hospitals. At Palermo, on the other hand, the ratio takes the values 1.57, 1.45, 1.40, 1.28 and 1.14, respectively, for births taking place at home, at the University Hospital, at Public Hospital A, at Public Hospital B and in the private clinics. The last of these results suggests that different conventions may have been applied at the private clinics, but some form of population selection may also have been involved.

The main conclusion which can be drawn from these results is that, even in the most favourable circumstances, attempts to differentiate between late fetal and early neonatal deaths may be unrealistic. In consequence, the use of perinatal mortality rate as a measure of the adequacy of maternity care (in preference to the separate late fetal and early neonatal rates from which it is constructed) is to be recommended. Furthermore, in the calculation of mortality rates, a denominator formed by the total of live births is probably less reliable than one formed by the total of live births and late fetal deaths. This is of course an implicit criticism of the conventional procedure for computing infant mortality rates.

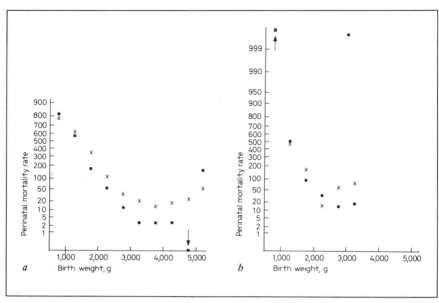

Fig. 1. Perinatal mortality and birth weight in single (a) and twin (b) births. x = Palermo; • = Göteborg.

A salient feature of both surveys is the marked variation of mortality in terms of maturity, as represented by birth weight. Overall mortality in a population reflects to a considerable extent the distribution of maturity. If the levels of mortality in two populations are compared, due account must be taken of the distribution of maturity if the full significance of the results is to be revealed. The position is analogous to the comparison of mortality rates in general populations (i.e. covering all age groups). In this situation, the need to standardise mortality rates to compensate for differences in age and sex is now widely accepted and the time is surely ripe for extending the same device to comparisons of perinatal, neonatal and infant mortality rates. When an indicator of maturity is chosen to form the basis of such a standardisation procedure, it would in theory be desirable to consider a variety of measurements. In practice, however, most suitable indicators would not be obtained unless special techniques were to be employed for data collection. The most readily available and reliable single indicator of maturity is birth weight, and birth weight provides an effective basis for standardisation.

The relationship between perinatal mortality and birth weight is illustrated in figure 1a and b, which refer respectively to single and twin births. In these figures, the perinatal mortality rates have been plotted on a non-uniform 'probability' or 'probit' scale. Scales of this kind are commonly used in the presentation of the results of biological assays of drugs, the objective being to express the relation between the proportion of organisms showing the characteristic response and the applied dosage in a linear form. Reference to figure 1a shows that the mortality-birth weight relationship may be divided naturally into three parts. For birth weights of up to about 3,000 g, mortality falls linearly with increasing birth weight, from a level of 800–900 per 1,000 to below 20 per 1,000. This is the classical form of relation found in biological assay. It indicates that, at a given birth weight, what might be termed the 'susceptibilities' of the infants belonging to the particular population follow a normal or Gaussian distribution, whose variance is constant throughout the range of birth weights. Between 3,000 and 5,000 g birth weight, the mortality rate remains at a low and relatively stable level (any differences are magnified by the probit scale). The third part of the relationship covers birth weights of above about 5,000 g, for which the mortality rate tends to be substantially higher than in the 3,000–5,000-gram part of the range. On general grounds, it is apparent that the three parts of the relation correspond to three separate sets of clinical problems. When describing perinatal mortality in a population, each of the three parts should be considered separately, and there is no *a priori* reason why trends in one part should be accompanied by corresponding trends in another part of the scale. When the two surveys are compared the perinatal mortality rates are similar for birth weights of below 1,500 g. However, the rate of decrease of mortality with increasing birth weight is greater at Göteborg, so much so that when the 'plateau' between 3,000 and 4,000 g is reached, the mortality rate is less than a quarter of that at Palermo.

Reference to figure 1b shows that the perinatal mortality-birth weight relation for twins is of a similar form to that for single births. However, the 'plateau' is reached at a birth weight of 2,000 g. Comparison of figures 1a and b shows that for birth weights of between 1,500 and 2,500 g, the perinatal mortality rate for twins is lower than that for single births, whereas for birth weigths of above 2,500 g the mortality rate for twins is substantially higher. Mortality is higher at Palermo than at Göteborg for the whole range of birth weights below 3,500 g, which cover almost all the twin births.

In the absence of detailed data about birth weights, a simpler, but nevertheless very useful, device is to divide the births into two parts, depending upon whether the birth weight is less than or greater than or equal to 2,500 g. The 2,500-gram birth weight is well established in the literature as a realistic boundary between 'low weight' and 'higher weight' births. In this way, for single births the below 2,500-gram group corresponds largely to the first of the three parts of the perinatal mortality-birth weight relationship, whilst the 2,500-gram and above group largely reflects the second part, since the proportion of births weighing 5,000 g or more is very small. This form of analysis is illustrated in

Table VI. Perinatal mortality in terms of place of delivery, multiplicity and birth weight groups: rate per 1,000 live and still births

Place of delivery	Birth weight, g			
	below 2,501 g		2,501 g and above	
	single births	twins	single births	twins
Göteborg				
West Hospital	196	306	4	18
East Hospital	160	115	4	13
Both	178	185	4	15
Palermo				
University Hospital	339	111	32	235
Public Hospital A	340	292	50	0
Public Hospital B	333	273	31	59
Public Hospital A or B	318	0	42	250
Private clinic	164	120	9	21
Home	178	0	12	0
All	235	160	20	59

table VI, which shows perinatal mortality in the under 2,500-gram group and 2,500-gram and over birth weight group in terms of place of delivery. At Göteborg, mortality of low weight single births in the East Hospital is lower than that at the West Hospital. At Palermo, it is clear that the main difference between the three hospitals is in the mortality rate in the 2,500-gram and above birth weight group. The results for twins reflect the differences between places of confinement noted for single births, are based upon relatively small numbers and should be treated with reserve.

The surveys have confirmed our original belief that there might be large variations in mortality rates between the two cities. In almost every respect Palermo is at a disadvantage, and particularly in terms of late fetal deaths. It is interesting that the relative difference in mortality rates is greatest in those parts of the birth weight distribution for which absolute levels of mortality are least. Amongst those sections of the population, such as low weight, single births and twins, which might on general grounds be expected to reflect better technical facilities and more advanced medical practice, the relative differences between the two surveys are lowest. In terms of reducing mortality, it is clear that to concentrate upon the 3,000–4,500-gram birth weight range at Palermo might be much more effective than the application of similar resources to, say, the low weight births. In particular, the better control of infection at Palermo might well be very effective in terms of lives saved, at comparatively little cost. We have found that the differences in mortality rates between the two cities cannot be attributed to differences in the distribution of birth weight. Other factors must be involved and the more detailed analysis reported in the remainder of the supplement will help to identify the role of maternal characteristics, past obstetric history, socio-economic conditions and other matters about which data have been collected.

On both surveys, there were significant variations in reported mortality between the various places of confinement. At Göteborg, these appear to be due in part to variations in the conventions used for differentiating between late fetal deaths and deaths immediately following live births. At Palermo, the variations were much greater, but there is little doubt that population selection must have played some part. This factor will be examined in detail in subsequent analyses.

This introductory section, while going deeper than the traditional approach to such surveys of perinatal and infant mortality is, nevertheless, general; in some respect, masking important significant findings. These can only be gleaned after going into more depth and using sophisticated biometric techniques. In the sections that follow, this point will become apparent and serve as an indication of how care must be taken in the interpretation of traditional more general data.

References

Ashford, J.R.: Epidemiological and biometric issues in infant mortality; in *Falkner* Key issues in infant mortality. Report of a conference, Washington 1969 (National Institutes of Child Health and Human Development, Bethesda 1970).

Ashford, J.R.; Fryer, J.G., and Brimblecombe, F.S.W.: Secular trends in late foetal deaths, neonatal mortality and birthweight in England and Wales 1956–65. Br. J. prev. Soc. Med. *23:* 154–162 (1969).

Brimblecombe, F.S.W.; Ashford, J.R., and Fryer, J.G.: Significance of low birthweight in perinatal mortality. Br. J. prev. Soc. Med. *22:* 27–35 (1968).

Prof. *J.R. Ashford,* Department of Mathematical Statistics and Operational Research, University of Exeter, *Exeter EX4 4PU* (England)

Section II

Monogr. Paediat., vol. 9, pp. 24–32 (Karger, Basel 1977)

Monitoring Perinatal Information – A Medical Birth Record

P. Karlberg, U. Selstam and T. Landström

Department of Pediatrics I, University of Göteborg, Göteborg

Background

Birth, the transfer from intrauterine life as a fetus to extrauterine life as a newborn infant, represents the most important change of environment in an individual's life.

The process of labor and delivery entails in itself mechanical and functional strains on the fetus. The exposure to the new external surroundings, with the demands of functional independence, requires an adaptation of most body functions. The outcome depends on the relationship between the strength of these external factors and the capacity of the fetus/newborn infant to cope with the situation, i.e. the condition of the fetus prior to initiation of parturition. This condition of the fetus depends on several factors: (1) fetal age, i.e. gestational duration; (2) fetal growth and development – stage of normal growth and development pattern; fetopathy caused by disturbance during the second and third trimesters; embryopathy, caused by disturbances during the first trimester; (3) chromosomal abnormality and genetic disorders. Many of these factors are interrelated.

Most results of early damage during intrauterine life will not be discovered until after birth, and they may have no functional significance before this, i.e. they increase the hazards of the neonatal period. The outcome may be spontaneous abortion, stillbirth or live birth. The latter is differentiated in early neonatal death, late neonatal death, irreversible damage with sequelae, intact survival after transient disturbances or intact survival after an uneventful course. Thus, the period around birth – the perinatal period – is of essential importance for the individual life span.

Need for Monitoring Perinatal Information

Information on the perinatal course, and related factors, is of interest from several points of view: for cases of perinatal survival, in connection with health care contacts during infancy, childhood and adolescence; in the event of perinatal death for medical advice to the parents and as guidance for perinatal management of subsequent pregnancies and deliveries, and treatment of newborn infants; for analysis of associated risk-factors and possibly related etiological factors; for analysis of the effect of perinatal care; for analyses of biological mechanisms and processes; for obtaining pointers in the design of specially directed studies; for analysis of the origin of subsamples selected for special studies; for epidemiological studies; for improvement of vital statistics and hospital statistics, and for identification of priorities for improvement of perinatal care.

The goal is to minimize the risks during passage across the perinatal period by preventive measures, and effective treatment of disturbances. The spin-off effect is a more rational utilization of available resources for perinatal care.

Aim of the Present Work

The aim of the present work is to develop a perinatal information system which meets several of the above requirements and which is suitable for routine clinical use. The information should be summarized and concentrated on a single sheet of paper, presented in a form directly readable and useful to the clinician, and at the same time suitable as a basis for computerization. To emphasize the expected clinical applicability of the system the information for each case is called the *medical birth record.*

Development of the Medical Birth Record

The work started in 1968 at the Deparment of Pediatrics, University of Göteborg, with a preliminary study. The fact that in Sweden practically all deliveries take place in hospitals and around three quarters in hospitals with obstetric and pediatric departments has had a direct influence on the structure of the system.

Göteborg, the second largest city in Sweden, with half a million inhabitants, has two maternity hospitals and one children's hospital. In each maternity hospital there is a neonatal unit supervised by the Department of Pediatrics, including the general care of all newborn infants born in the hospital. There are around 3,000 deliveries per annum in each hospital. A test study was performed at one of the maternity units, the University Department of Gynaecology and Obstetrics, Sahlgrenska sjukhuset. The information system has been in operation there since 1970.

A working group of obstetricians, midwives, pediatricians, nurses and administrators, appointed by the National Board of Health and Welfare and chaired by one of us (P.K.), started in 1971 to explore the possibilities of introducing the system generally in Sweden. Since 1973, it is in operation at all maternity hospitals, thus also at the second maternity hospital in Göteborg. A retrospective introduction from hospital records was, however, performed for 1972.

Data 'Botanization'

A systematized information procedure requires a selection of meaningful variables, i.e. possibly useful in clinical synthesis, epidemiological analyses and/or hypothesis-testing, and which can be described, classified, and coded. We call this basic work data 'botanization'. A general rule has also to be considered: a large number of items demands a limited number of cases; a large number of cases demands a limited number of items. Such work must be based on a series of clinical, methodological, and epidemiological judgements, taking different judgements into consideration. In the development of the system, several versions have been tested. The version presented and discussed here has been used since 1973.

Data Content

The perinatal information selected is recorded under the following main headings (appendix 3).

Identification, including maternal and paternal age, marital status.

Previous obstetrical history. Number of pregnancies, stillbirths, live births, neonatal deaths. Time since last birth.

Current pregnancy. Last menstrual period (LMP), date of first day. Antenatal care: yes/no. Optionally: number of visits, time of first visit. Complications.

Delivery. Mode of delivery, anaesthesia, intervention, complications. Puerperal complications.

Newborn infant. Time of birth. Single or multiple, with order of birth. Sillbirth before/during labour or live birth. Apgar score: 1 min, 5 min. Birth size: weight, length, head circumference.

Neonatal course. Mainly clinical diagnoses. Optionally: degree, severity.

Neonatal treatment. Any specific treatment. Optionally: duration when applicable.

Discharge. Time. Condition: alive to home, to other unit, to other department, or dead. Autopsy: yes/no. Planned health control.

Clinical Conditions and Intervention

Clinical conditions and intervention measures are classified according to the Swedish adaptation of the 1965 version of the ICD (International Statistical Classification of Diseases, Injuries and Causes of Death) and the Swedish classification of operations and other forms of intervention specified by the National Board of Health and Welfare. By law, these two classifications are to be used for the annual reports of activities at all Swedish hospitals.

The Swedish adaptation of the ICD differs from the original version by having a more detailed specification of subcategories. The principle has been to keep the digits in the ICD unchanged and designate the further specification by a fifth digit. In the adaptation of the version used it was possible to include several perinatal diagnoses that were missed clinically. In the latest version of the classification of operations and other forms of intervention, which utilized a fourth coding digit, it was also possible to carry out supplemental adaptations for perinatal clinical activity.

In order to facilitate and systematize the classification, the most commonly recorded diagnoses and intervention measures were arranged in clinically appropriate order, called 'oribs' or 'lazy dog'. In addition to the verbal description, applicable code numbers were given.

The combined diagnoses between obstetrical events and neonatal disturbances, No. 764–768 in the ICD, and also in the Swedish version, are excluded. A more detailed specification will be obtained with separated diagnoses.

Separated diagnoses:
657 Delivery complicated by prolonged labor with subgroups.
772 Birth injury without mention of cause with subgroups.
Combined diagnoses:
767 Difficult labor with abnormality forces of labor without obstetrical subgroups and only main neonatal morbidity groups.

After the obstetrician has described maternal/obstetrical events and the pediatrician, the neonatal ones, any significant influences of various maternal/obstetrical factors on the neonatal course may be recorded, either as 'yes' or 'no', or on a graduated scale when possible – likely or definite influence. The severity of the various neonatal conditions may also be graded on a three-point scale.

Procedure

Working protocols for hospital records – one for antenatal care, one for labor and delivery and one for newborn infants – have been designed for clinical recording of basic information in an easily recognizable fashion. The sheet for newborn babies (also used in applicable parts for stillbirths) is shown in appendices 4 and 5. The front contains the basic information and enough space for clinical examinations in fairly uneventful cases; in more complicated cases, extra sheets are used. Discharge notes are placed at the end. The reverse of the sheet contains the diagnosis items.

The information from the different forms is transferred by the secretary to the medical birth record form. Numerical variables are written or typed directly in specified places and verbal descriptions in specified sections (appendices 6 and 7). The completed form is then checked by the obstetrician and by the pediatrician. Relationsships between maternal/obstetrical and neonatal events are evaluated and recorded. The individual medical birth record is then complete.

Distribution

The medical birth record is prepared in one original and three copies. The original record serves as the first page of the hospital record. Copy 1 is sent to the child health clinic for each individual infant. Copy 2 is sent to the Antenatal Clinic for information at the post-natal follow-up. Copy 3 is used for local/ regional/central computerized analyses.

Discussion

There is an obvious need for individual perinatal information for several purposes. The requirements vary, however, according to the intended purpose. The present work has been based on the principle that there is certain basic information that is required for all purposes. In order to avoid repeated recordings, a systematized perinatal data base is developed to which further structured information may be added in a modular fashion. In the literature, several designs for perinatal information systems, using variable sets of forms and items have been described. The information system presented here is based on currently available information within the perinatal health care system. The extraction of information has been systematized and facilitated by structuring clinical working protocols. Clinical assessments, such as diagnosis of diseases and disorders, and descriptions of clinical intervention, are included in structural form. An information system of this type will consist of data of differing character — 'hard', 'soft' and varying degrees in between.

The character of each data item must be borne in mind in any subsequent analyses. This means that the information system makes demands on the user. The key factors for any information system, the data 'botanization' — selection, classification, codification — is discussed in this context.

Items of a Basic Character

Items generally considered as basic and clearly defineable will be included in any kind of information system without debate. In the case of the present system, these include: identification of the mother and/or newborn infant, maternal age, and place of confinement. Concerning the newborn infant: date of birth, birth weight, single or multiple, order of birth, alive or not, and surviving 7 days, possibly 21 days, or not. Extra items that may be included are parental age and marital status.

Gestational age is a vital basic item. With known LMP and birth date it is easily calculated. Should it then be corrected to 4 weeks interval between the menstrual periods in the cases with longer or shorter intervals? There is, in any case, always a risk of misinterpretation of the last menstrual flow as being one menstruation too late or too early. The use of oral contraceptives has increased this difficulty. Should the calculation also be based on early antenatal obstetrical examination? Should it be supplemented or, alternatively, be based on a pediatric neonatal examination?

In our opinion, there is only one way to proceed: We calculate from a known LMP a basic gestational age (GA). If LMP is not known, basic GA is recorded as *not known.* Supplementary information used: Interval length between menstrual periods. Extra information: separately recorded obstetrical GA and pediatric GA. If the recorded GA is primarily based on a weighing of these three assessments, subsequent analyses will be less accurate, and there will be a risk of masking clinically important biological relationships.

Measures of size of the newborn infant, apart from birth weight, such as length and head circumference, are of increasing interest, especially in relation to GA and to each other. Accuracy should increase if these measurements are performed a few days postnatally, due to the possible increased muscular tone and head molding at birth, but this will often introduce practical difficulties. Also, there will be a risk of missing measurements. We have chosen to include length and head circumference at birth with optional inclusion of values after a few days (separately recorded).

Although birth weight is rarely unrecorded, it will realistically, take some time before length and head circumference are recorded routinely in all cases.

Parity is another basic item of great interest. It forms a part of the *previous obstetrical history* and further information is wanted in most analyses, e.g. number of stillbirths and number of early neonatal deaths. We have, for the sake of simplicity, chosen the number of stillbirths, live births and early neonatal deaths, which means that earlier multiple births will introduce an error in the calculation of parity (stillbirths + live births).

Birth weight and also gestational age for each previous birth are certainly desirable for several analyses but have been excluded in order to limit the numbers of items.

The number of pregnancies is of interest as the difference between this and parity equals the number of abortions. However, this item will always have a varying quality, since the number of early miscarriages will be recorded with varying accuracy. Late abortion, spontaneous and medically induced, is of definite interest. In making up a medical birth record for general use and central analysis, it was decided, in order to preserve the personal integrity of the mother, that no definite distinctions should be made. The number of pregnancies is thus clearly 'soft' data, the method used for calculation of parity also contributing to this. In the next version, this point may be defined more precisely.

Mode of delivery. Basic information in this connection clearly includes the following: (1) Vaginal delivery. Preferably supplement information: spontaneous, forceps, vacuum extractor and induction. (2) Presentation: vertex, breech or other. (3) Cesarean section. Preferably supplement information: elective or emergency. Desirable further items of high priority include indications for any intervention measures performed, and also the presence of certain specific maternal diseases or disorders, such as diabetes or toxicosis, is important.

The condition of the newborn infant immediately after birth is another basic item of information. Scoring according to Apgar has now been used in practice so extensively that the Apgar score at 1 and 5 min is considered useful.

Neonatal course. Apart from death, transfer to another unit or department is an objective item, as also is the duration of any special treatment. Taking into account that the implications of such items will depend on the resources and practical rules applied at the time, such items are considered to be valuable and fairly 'hard'.

Other desirable items of high priority are significant morbidity and causes of death, such as malformations of functional significance, respiratory disorders, circulatory disorders, hemolytic disease, infections, metabolic diseases, etc. In this connection, the requirements will be unlimited, as is also the case concerning complications during pregnancy and delivery.

A detailed clinical perinatal course, including basic and extra information is also desirable. Some questions come readily to mind: Should objective examinations and laboratory findings be recorded, or only a summarized clinical evaluation and the degree of severity of a diagnosed condition? Such a recording, however, requires a detailed description and definitions to be evenly 'hard'. For example: toxicosis and hyaline membrane disease in newborn infants are two frequently recorded diagnoses, but are not always easy to differentiate in the individual patient.

In the perinatal information system presented, the diagnosis and clinical intervention are accepted as a basis for analysis of the perinatal course. They form part of the clinical work and are used for clinical communication at the next contact with the patient by the primary doctor, or by a doctor to whom the patient is referred. They are also used in the official hospital statistics. Thus, in order to utilize the medical birth record for communication within the health care system and for hospital records, diagnoses and any intervention must be included. The quality of such data will vary between centers, and also within centers, and must generally be considered as 'soft'. However, some items, for instance maternal diabetes, are 'hard', and it is possible to tighten up the diagnostic routines locally, regionally, nationally, and internationally. At present, a working group within the Swedish Research Council is exploring the possibility of introducing a system of differentiation for respiratory disorders in newborn infants applicable to the whole country. However, it is obviously not an easy task and will take time. In the meantime, clinical diagnosis and clinical intervention, if analyzed with care, can provide important information (section IV of this volume).

Other Items of Medical and Social Significance

Antenatal care has been given great emphasis in most perinatal information surveys. It involves many factors, however, and must be related to the local system of health care. In Sweden, lack of antenatal care is regarded as a sign of inability to organize one's life or, at the other extreme, a strong desire to remain outside the arrangements of the community. A high number of visits to an antenatal clinic may indicate medical problems, or risks, or maternal anxiety. In the medical birth record presented here, the information content is kept low, on the assumption that significant situations will turn up in the clinical diagnosis. Smoking habits and alcohol habits have been considered for inclusion, but it was decided to omit them. To be able to include them in a meaningful way, special studies with special resources are required.

Social factors, such as the mother's and father's education, occupation, and social class, and the mother's employment before and during pregnancy are certainly of interest, but have been left out since they also require special studies. The need for information for the evaluation of social risk groups, not only for pregnancy but also for newborn infants and their development, is obvious. Working groups are currently tackling these problems.

Practical Experience

The perinatal information system has been in operation since 1970 in Göteborg and since 1973 in the whole country. As in all information systems, there is a need for continuous checking of the data collected. If the original information recorded in the working protocol of the hospital records can be extracted directly for computer processing, the transformation into data banks will be facilitated. Primary checking of the data will then be achieved more quickly and with greater accuracy and motivation, and the printout of the information for distribution will be obtained as a byproduct. Trials are in progress and test runs have been carried out. Built-in computerized checking systems are under development. The present study is one validation study and validation studies have also started for the whole country. To date, the number of births and number of deaths are practically identical with official vital statistics.

Summary

The need for systematized perinatal information for each newborn infant for the health care of each individual as well as for epidemiological, biomedical, clinical, and administrative analysis is stressed.

A system of monitoring perinatal information, called the medical birth record, which forms a part of the clinical work, is presented. It is concentrated on a single sheet and has several applications. The clinical classification and coding are based on the Swedish adaptation of ICD, with more detailed specification of subcategories.

The quality of items used is discussed, and the differences in 'hardness' of the various items are pointed out. Such differences are present in all clinical information systems and must be accepted, but it is essential to be aware of these differences and take them into account when planning analyses and interpreting the results.

Prof. *P. Karlberg,* Department of Pediatrics, University of Göteborg, East Hospital, *Göteborg S–416 85* (Sweden)

Section III

Monogr. Paediat., vol. 9, pp. 33–85 (Karger, Basel 1977)

Some Indicators of Maturity

J.G. Fryer, R.A. Harding, J.R. Ashford and P. Karlberg

Department of Mathematical Statistics and Operational Research, University of Exeter, Exeter, Devon

I. Introduction

Although there is no generally agreed definition of the term 'mature' as applied to new-born infants, there is widespread acceptance of a number of indicators of maturity. Since it is universally agreed that the 'maturity' of an infant directly or indirectly exerts a considerable influence on its experiences after delivery (and before, for that matter), it follows that in any wide-ranging perinatal survey, and especially in comparative ones such as ours, information on these 'indicators' of maturity should be collected and analyzed. The purpose of this paper is simply to present a preliminary descriptive statistical analysis of the data that we have collected in Palermo and Göteborg. Most of what we have to say about these indicators and their associations with other factors will be found in this section, but an analysis of the all-important mortality-maturity relationships is delayed until paper 5.

The most commonly recorded indicator of the maturity of an infant in routine statistics is its birth weight. Although this characteristic is indicative of other things than 'maturity', it is relatively simple to measure accurately and has a key role to play. Gestational age, the time-dependent indicator, is less commonly recorded partly because it is often much more difficult to assess accurately. We include an extensive account of both of these characteristics in this section, singly and jointly. Crown-heel length is another generally recognized indicator of maturity that we have covered, though this too is considerably more difficult to assess than birth weight. Finally, for Göteborg but not Palermo, we have information on head circumference, another characteristic which is not simple to measure consistently. Of course, many other acceptable indicators exist, both physical and otherwise, but the line has to be drawn somewhere and, for better or for worse, we have concentrated our efforts on these four. Presumably most people would consider them to be among the most sensitive. These four indicators are quite strongly associated with each other, but each has a somewhat different story to tell. Jointly, they may well exhaust most of the information to be gained from any wider set of maturity indicators.

II. Birth Weight

Although in principle birth weight is simple to determine accurately (in our surveys it is formally recorded to the nearest 10 g), in practice it is often rounded to the nearest attractively simple number (like 2,500 g). This 'digit preference' is common and may be bothersome depending on the use to be made of the information. It is the distribution of birth weight over all or part of the population which seems to us to be the most natural and useful summary of the individual birth weights. This simultaneously characterizes the location and spread of frequency or probability and provides estimates of parameters like median birth weight and other percentage points. However, in the face of strong digit preference, we need to be careful when choosing boundary points of birth weight groups, since otherwise strong bias in our estimates will result. Digit preference shows up more clearly in the Palermo data than it does in the data from Göteborg. For example, in the birth weight groups 2,351–2,400, 2,401–2,450, 2,451–2,500, 2,501–2,550 and 2,551–2,600 g, Palermo shows frequencies of 59, 16, 106, 12 and 78, respectively, whilst the corresponding numbers for Göteborg are 40, 47, 60, 74 and 75. Allowing values like 2,500 g to be end-points when cumulating the distribution of birth weight for Palermo simply produces highly upward-biased estimates of the cumulative distribution at those points (and this is probably true of much birth weight data reported elsewhere). So we have instead used end-points like 2,375 g and 2,625 g which are less affected by digit preference, and a group width generally of 250 g (in order to give plots a relatively smooth appearance). Interpolation can then be used to gain a more accurate assessment of the distribution at points in between, like 2,500 g, if these are of particular interest.

The overall cumulative distributions of birth weight for the two cities by multiplicity of birth are plotted on a probit scale in figure 1. The numbers on which these plots (and others) are based are summarized in tables I–III. In most cases, but not all, the proportions of 'unknowns' for Göteborg are low. This is not true of the *total survey* data for Palermo, however. Naturally, whenever missing percentages are relatively low, we base our plots on the total survey data. When this is not the case (for example when we are dealing with birth length or gestational age) we make use of the sample selected from all infants with standard records (appendix 2, section VII), though missing percentages here are somewhat high on occasion. Standard errors of the plotted estimates of the *true* cumulative distribution are given on the graphs to provide a base for making

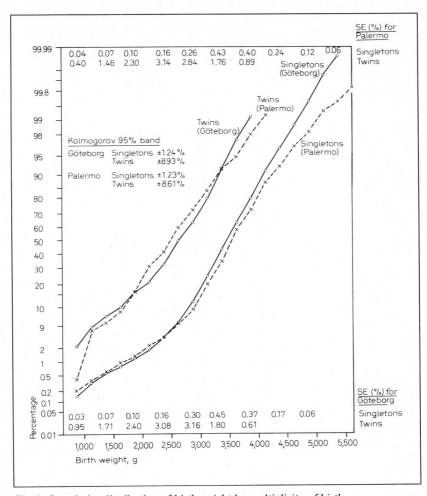

Fig. 1. Cumulative distribution of birth weight by multiplicity of birth.

comparisons on a point-by-point basis, and they are placed above or below the plotted point to which they refer. Also included is the width of the 95% 'Kolmogorov Band', which provides a confidence region for the whole cumulative distribution function. So for a 95% confidence region for the cumulative distribution function of birth weight of Göteborg singletons, for example, simply draw a band of half-width 1.24% about the sample cumulative curve. In a long sequence of such trials, 95 out of 100 bands will almost certainly cover the *true* distribution function in its entirety.

Table I. Further details on cumulative distributions of birth weight

Factor	Number (and percentage) of infants unclassified and their perinatal mortality rate	Sub-population within factor	Number of infants in sub-population (and percentage of total classified)	Number of infants of unknown birth weight in sub-population	Percentage unknown in sub-population	Perinatal mortality rate for total sub-population	infants of unknown birth weight in sub-population
(a) Göteborg							
Multiplicity	none —	singletons twins others	12,039 (98.1) 232 (1.9) 3 (0.0)	zero zero zero	zero zero zero	11.4 86.2 zero	— — —
Sex	none —	male female	6,061 (50.3) 5,978 (49.7)	zero zero	zero zero	13.5 9.2	— —
Outcome	none —	perinatal deaths survivors	137 (1.1) 11,902 (98.9)	zero zero	zero zero	— —	— —
Maternal age years	none —	less than 20 20–34 35 and more	653 (5.4) 10,669 (88.6) 717 (6.0)	zero zero zero	zero zero zero	13.8 10.7 19.5	— — —
Parity	none —	parity 0 1 and 2 3 and more	6,146 (51.1) 5,282 (43.9) 611 (5.1)	zero zero zero	zero zero zero	12.0 8.7 27.8	— — —
Complications of pregnancy	none —	complications no complications	5,061 (42.0) 6,978 (58.0)	zero zero	zero zero	15.2 11.0	— —

(b) Palermo

Factor							
Multiplicity	none	singletons	12,910 (97.9)	622	4.8	33.2	83.6
	—	twins	266 (2.0)	17	6.4	124.1	352.9
		others	12 (0.1)	3	25.0	500.0	zero
Sex	260 (2.0)	male	6,467 (51.1)	198	3.1	36.6	136.4
	30.8	female	6,183 (48.9)	202	3.3	29.8	89.1
Outcome	none	perinatal deaths	429 (3.3)	52	12.1	—	—
		survivors	12,481 (96.7)	570	4.6	—	—
Maternal age years	434 (3.4)	less than 20	1,256 (10.1)	31	2.5	25.5	32.3
	106.0	20–34	9,485 (76.0)	257	2.7	26.0	31.1
		35 and more	1,735 (13.9)	55	3.2	59.9	90.9
Parity*	36 (0.8)	parity 0	1,724 (37.3)	22	1.3	26.1	136.4
	83.3	1 and 2	1,998 (43.2)	44	2.2	22.0	45.5
		3 and more	898 (19.4)	43	4.8	63.5	46.5
Social class*	10 (0.2)	1, 2	614 (13.2)	9	1.5	19.5	111.1
	zero	3	2,686 (57.8)	64	2.4	29.8	78.1
		4, 5	810 (17.4)	25	3.1	37.0	zero
		0	512 (11.0)	16	3.1	50.8	38.5
		other	24 (0.5)	zero	zero	41.7	zero

Notes which apply here and equally to similar tables: (1) factors marked with an asterisk use the ESR sample; (2) all cases refer to singletons unless stated otherwise; (3) perinatal mortality rate is rate per 1,000 births.

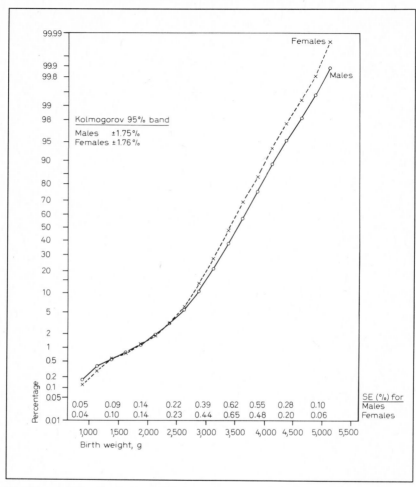

2a

Fig. 2. Cumulative distribution of birth weight of singletons by sex in Göteborg (a) and Palermo (b).

Among singletons, the proportions of low weight infants appears to be similar in the two cities, which is not what we had expected to find. Beyond 2,500 g the two plots begin to diverge with Göteborg showing an excess of 8% by 3,375 g or so. This gap continues as birth weight increases further, Palermo showing a very long upper tail. In reaching this conclusion, however, we need to bear in mind two further things. Firstly, 4.8% of all birth weights from Palermo are 'unknown', these showing a perinatal mortality rate of 83.6 per 1,000 births compared with the rate of 33.2 per 1,000 for Palermo as a whole. So the lower

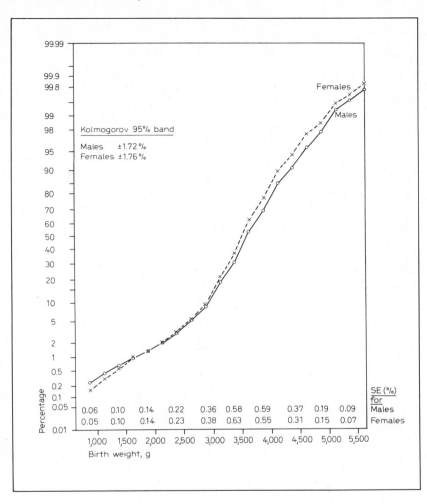

2b

tail of the distribution plotted in figure 1 almost certainly underestimates the true proportion of low weight infants in Palermo to some extent. This means that whilst we can confidently say that median birth weights for the two cities differ by only 100 g or so, we cannot make really *precise* comparisons between the proportions of low-weight infants. Secondly, some of the birth weights from Palermo were measured and recorded some days after the time of delivery and this might account in part for the behaviour in the upper tail. However, as we shall see later on, gestational ages tend to contradict this since they also show a long upper tail. The corresponding cumulatives for twins in figure 1 show a somewhat different pattern, but they are based on relatively small numbers and consequently have much larger standard errors. Differences between the two cumulatives rarely exceed two standard errors.

Comparing the forms of these two cumulatives for singletons visually with those that we have encountered previously (*Brimblecombe et al.,* 1968, for example), in other populations, we find that whilst Göteborg conforms the position of Palermo is less clear. Its behaviour from 3,750 g onward does not appear to be typical of patterns that we have seen in British and US data. This impression is further supported by some tentative fitting of mathematical models to the birth weight data that we have carried out. We have noted previously that as a working approximation, the distribution of birth weight conforms qualitatively to a mixture of two Gaussian or normal components, rather than just one (the cumulative of which appears as a straight line on a probit scale). A large proportion of infants (90–95%) belong to a major or primary component with mean about 3,500 g and standard deviation 500 g or so. The rest make up a minor or secondary component with mean 2,000–2,500 g and standard deviation 700 g or thereabouts. The fit of this model typically improves considerably after some truncation of the upper tail of the distribution. Using the whole range and introducing a third component, much more than proportionately improves the fit as a rule. This third component, which has a relatively small standard deviation, is sited in the upper tail with a mean of 4,500 g or so, and typically contains only a very small percentage of the infants (1% at most). Preliminary fits of these models to the Palermo/Göteborg data show that the Swedish data conforms but that taken *literally* the Palermo data is difficult to force into this pattern. This could mean that the models that we have been using need to be widened to cover what is possibly a less homogeneous population. There are other possible biomedical explanations which are discussed in section VI, but clearly further studies would be needed to resolve the point.

To see how this important maturity indicator varies with other factors, we have split the overall data in many different ways and have plotted the resulting cumulative curves. In figure 2, we show sex differences. Relative to each other the two sexes show a similar pattern in each city. We find about the same proportion of males as females in the low weights, with a slight but statistically insignificant excess of males in the very lowest. Beyond 2,500 g or so, the proportions for females build up more quickly and by 3,750 g there is an excess of about 10% (two standard errors of the difference at that point is 1.7% or thereabouts). The shapes of the cumulatives for both males and females in the two cities are similar to the corresponding overall plots. In the case of Göteborg, the median weight for males is some 125 g higher than it is for females, the corresponding figure for Palermo being about 85 g.

Cumulatives of birth weight broken down by outcome of delivery and

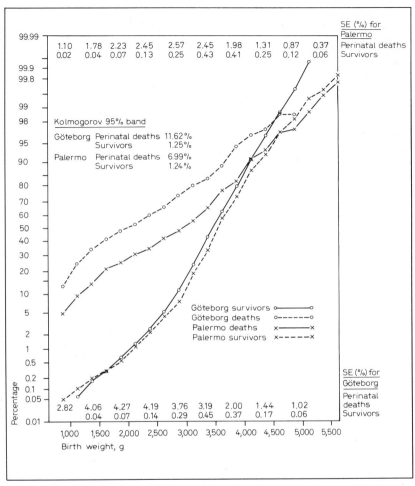

Fig. 3. Cumulative distribution of birth weight of singletons by outcome of birth.

shown in figure 3 are quite revealing. As anticipated, removing perinatal deaths lightens the lower tails of the distributions considerably. However, it is the cumulatives for perinatal deaths in the two cities which provide the really strik-ing feature. Taking the figures literally, we find that a much higher percentage of deaths in Göteborg are of relatively low weight (however, 12% of the perinatal deaths in Palermo have unknown weights, so the difference between the two may well be exaggerated). For example, in Göteborg, 63% weigh 2,500 g or less, compared with little more than 38% in Palermo. Because the total numbers of

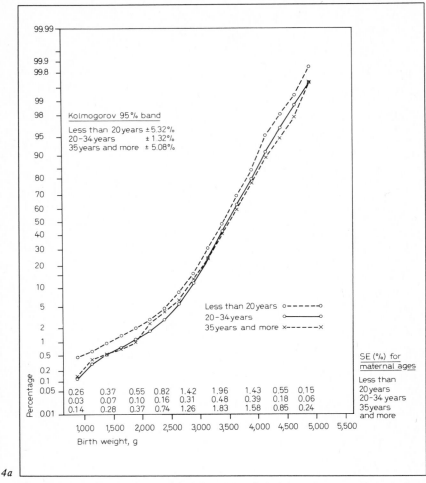

4a

Fig. 4. Cumulative distribution of birth weight of singletons by maternal age in Göteborg (a) and Palermo (b).

infants is of the same order of magnitude in the two cities in our survey and there are many more perinatal deaths in Palermo, it follows that birth weight-specific mortality rates for Göteborg must be considerably lower than those for Palermo for the most part beyond the lowest weights.

In figure 4, the data are broken down into three maternal age groups designed to contrast the behaviour of the centre with that of the two extremes. Table I shows that the distribution of maternal age in the two populations is quite different, Palermo having double the percentage in both the less than 20

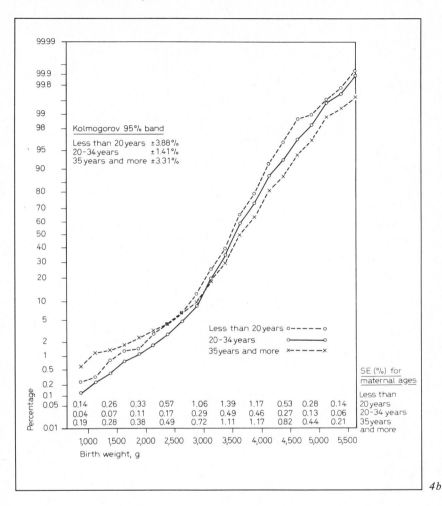

4b

years and 35 or more age groups, so the curves would need to be weighted differentially to compute the overall distribution. The discrepancy between the cumulative curves of the groups less than 20 years and 20–34 is considerable in both cities, the plot for young mothers lying consistently (and usually significantly) above that of the centre group so indicating lower weight. However, the behaviour of the 35 years or more group relative to the other two is really quite different. The distribution for Palermo, which is more extreme, shows heavy excesses in both tails (indicating larger variation) though this may be partly due

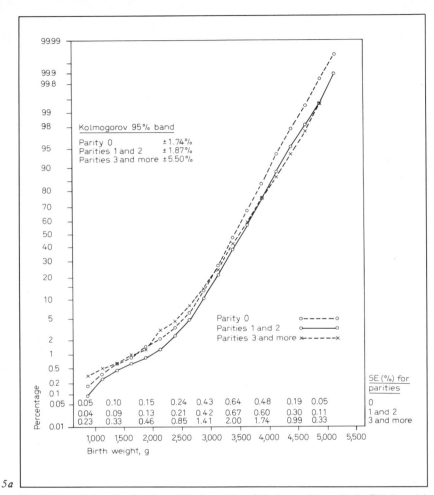

5a

Fig. 5. Cumulative distribution of birth weight of singletons by parity in Göteborg (a) and Palermo (b).

to the inclusion of mothers of advanced age (who are not present to the same extent in Göteborg). Even so, it is clear that the aberrant behaviour of the upper tail of the *overall* birth weight distribution for Palermo is not simply due to the presence of extreme maternal ages.

Figure 5 displays cumulatives for three parity groups, 0, 1 and 2 and 3 or more. Because of the large numbers of infants of unknown parity in the Palermo survey as a whole, we use the edited standard record (ESR) sample data here. As with maternal age, the distribution of parity is more extreme in Palermo, with

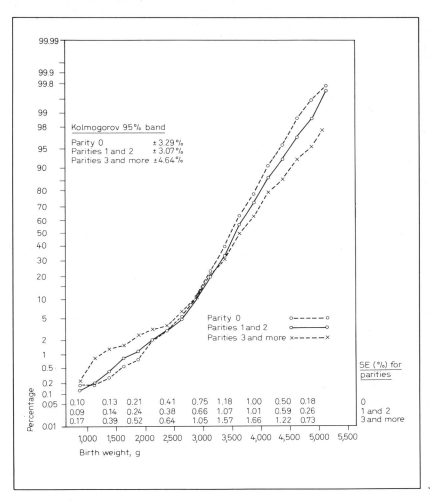

5b

20% or so of mothers in group 3 or more compared with 5% in Göteborg. The behaviour of the parity 3+ group in Palermo is qualitatively similar to that noted previously of maternal age group 35 years and more in that city. However, in Göteborg these two sub-populations seem to follow different patterns in the lowest weights. A further interesting feature of figure 5 is the contrast in the behaviour of parity 0 compared with parities 1 and 2 in the two cities among the lower birth weights. In the case of Göteborg, the cumulative for parity 0 lies entirely above that for 1 and 2 (indicating lower weight) and significantly so. By

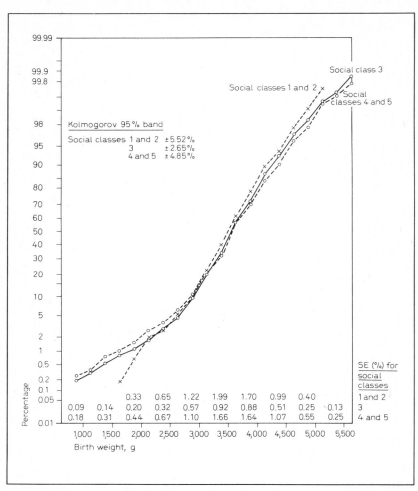

Fig. 6. Cumulative distribution of birth weight for Palermo singletons by social class of mother.

contrast, in sample form that for Palermo usually lies below, which is surprising. Although differences between the two curves for Palermo do not exceed two (pseudo) standard errors, the two cities do appear to follow different patterns in these two parity groups if we take the data literally.

Two further plots of cumulative birth weight have been included, one referring to Palermo only, the other to Göteborg. In figure 6, the Palermo data (again ESR) are broken down into three social class groups to produce meaningful curves. In figure 7, cumulatives are drawn on the basis of whether there were

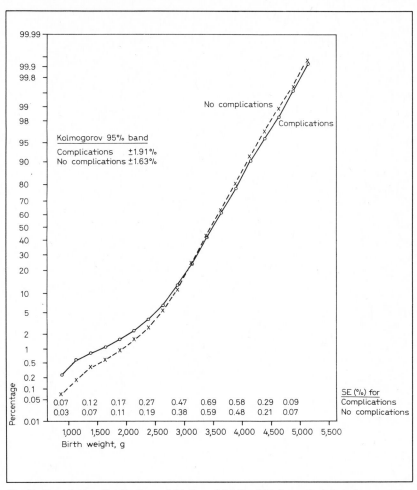

Fig. 7. Cumulative distribution of birth weight for Göteborg singletons by complications of pregnancy.

complications of pregnancy or not. These seem eminently reasonable too, and are very similar to those resulting from splitting the data by complications of delivery or not.

III. Gestational Age

The definition of gestational age used here is the standard one — the difference between the time of onset of the last menstrual period and the date of

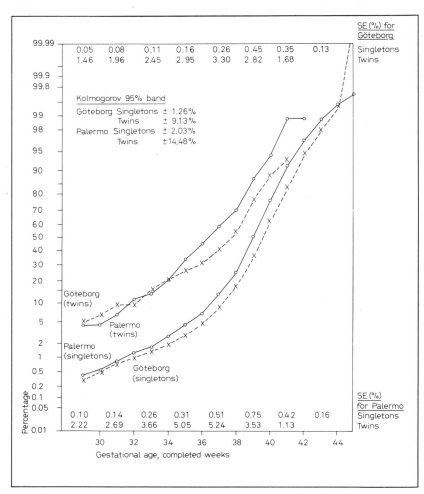

Fig. 8. Cumulative distributions of gestational age by multiplicity of birth.

delivery of the infant measured in *completed* weeks or days. All figures for Palermo are based on the ESR sample, since it was not recorded municipally. Figure 8, where the overall cumulatives for gestational age are displayed, shows some interesting patterns. Firstly, we ought to note that the cumulatives for Palermo singletons follows a similar trend to the corresponding plot for birth weight. Göteborg gestational ages also follow a similar trend to birth weight apart from the sharp cut-off at 44 weeks (probably due to curtailment of over-long pregnancies), which adds to the credibility of the mixture model. Secondly, relative to each other, these cumulatives show quite a different pattern compared with birth weight. They are similar in the very low gestational age region (though both may be underestimates), but from then on it is Palermo which cumulates more quickly, the two curves finally crossing only in the very high gestational ages. Judging by these data, the difference in the medians for the two cities is of the order of 4 days, the 'natural' gestational period being lower in Palermo. This gap widens to 6 days at the fifth percentile. However, we should note from table II that about 3.9% of the gestational ages in Göteborg are recorded as unknown, and have a perinatal mortality rate 50% higher than that of the survey as a whole. A slightly lower percentage is missing for Palermo, though these have a perinatal mortality rate of nearly 2.5 times the survey average. Both of these facts need to be borne in mind when assessing these data, and the non-random nature of the ESR sample should be noted. Apart from in the highest gestational ages, patterns for twins are qualitatively similar to those for singletons, but medians are some 2–3 weeks lower.

A further contrast between the two cities is provided by figure 9, where the data have been split by sex. In Göteborg, we find a higher percentage of males than females with low gestational age (differences frequently being much larger than two standard errors). However, the gap gradually narrows from 40 weeks onward and beyond 41 weeks the cumulatives are virtually coincident. The plots for Palermo, on the other hand, show an indecisive pattern for most of the range, differences being less than two standard errors, typically. However, there does seem to be an excess of males in the very high gestational ages. Both males and females in Palermo follow the overall trend for that city and likewise for Göteborg. Although we do not present the plots, on splitting the data by outcome of delivery we find much the same pattern as with birth weight, except that the contrast between the cumulatives for perinatal deaths is slightly less marked. However in both cities, but especially Palermo, the proportion of deaths with unknown gestational age has to be kept in mind.

Turning now to maternal age in figure 10, we see that in the initial part of the range the comparative behaviour of the three groups in Palermo is similar to that shown for birth weight, but that from then on (36 weeks or so) the differences are much less marked. Certainly, the cumulative for the 35 years or more group does not indicate a sizeable excess of infants with high gestational age compared with the other two groups. The cumulatives for Göteborg do not behave in a similar fashion to their birth weight counterparts, either. Apart from in the low gestational ages, the 35 years or more group leads the other two consistently with a median of 2 days less. Furthermore, among the lowest gestational ages, differences between the groups — less than 20 years and 20–34 are less marked than they are for birth weight and virtually coincide from 40 weeks onward. Especially because of the behaviour of the 35 years or more age group, we have to conclude again that Palermo and Göteborg show different patterns.

Table II. Further details on cumulative distributions of gestational age

Factor	Number (and percentage) of infants unclassified and their perinatal mortality rate	Sub-population within factor	Number of infants in sub-population (and percentage of total classified)	Number of infants of unknown gestational age in sub-population	Percentage unknown in sub-population	Perinatal mortality rate for	
						total sub-population	infants of unknown gestational age in sub-population
(a) Göteborg							
Multiplicity	none —	singletons twins others	12,039 (98.1) 232 (1.9) 3 (0.0)	467 10 zero	3.9 4.3 zero	11.4 86.2 zero	17.1 zero zero
Sex	none —	male female	6,061 (50.3) 5,978 (49.7)	206 261	3.4 4.4	13.5 9.2	4.9 26.8
Outcome	none —	perinatal deaths survivors	137 (1.1) 11,902 (98.9)	8 459	5.8 3.9	— —	— —
Maternal age years	none —	less than 20 20–34 35 and more	653 (5.4) 10,669 (88.6) 717 (6.0)	41 400 26	6.3 3.7 3.6	13.8 10.7 19.5	48.8 15.0 zero
Parity	none —	parity 0 1 and 2 3 or more	6,146 (51.1) 5,282 (43.9) 611 (5.1)	244 194 29	4.0 3.7 4.7	12.0 8.7 27.8	28.7 5.2 zero

(b) Palermo

Multiplicity*	none	–	singletons	4,656 (97.9)	168	3.6	32.0	77.4
			twins	93 (2.0)	5	5.4	107.5	200.0
			others	5 (0.1)	zero	zero	600.0	zero
Sex*	1 (0.02)	zero	male	2,374 (51.0)	79	3.3	33.7	101.3
			female	2,281 (49.0)	89	3.9	30.3	56.2
Outcome*	none	–	perinatal deaths	149 (3.2)	13	8.7	–	–
			survivors	4,507 (96.8)	155	3.4	–	–
Maternal age*	60 (1.3)	33.3	less than 20	520 (11.3)	26	5.0	28.8	zero
years			20–34	3,476 (75.6)	101	2.9	26.2	49.5
			35 and more	600 (13.1)	40	6.7	68.3	200.0
Parity*	36 (0.8)	83.3	parity 0	1,724 (37.3)	34	2.0	26.1	58.8
			1 and 2	1,998 (43.2)	61	3.1	22.0	32.8
			3 and more	898 (19.4)	67	7.5	63.5	119.4

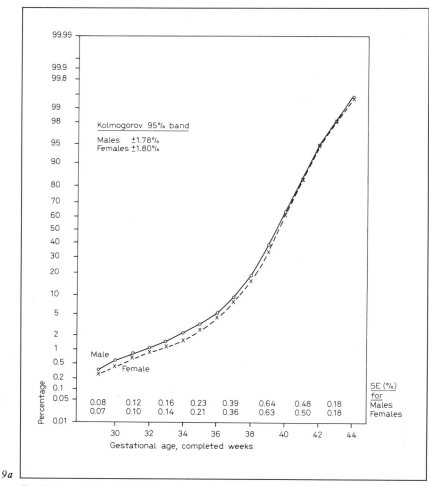

9a

Fig. 9. Cumulative distribution of gestational age of singletons by sex in Göteborg (a) and Palermo (b).

But we should not forget that the distribution of maternal age in the two cities over these three age groups (or within, either) is by no means identical.

As far as parity is concerned (fig. 11), the pattern for group 3 or more differs substantially from that of the other two groups in both Palermo and Göteborg. Although differences between groups 0 and 1 and 2 are relatively small in both cities, the Palermo sample cumulative for parity 0 lags that of 1 and 2 almost everywhere, often significantly, so indicating higher gestational age. This is also true for Göteborg beyond 39 weeks, but for lower gestational ages

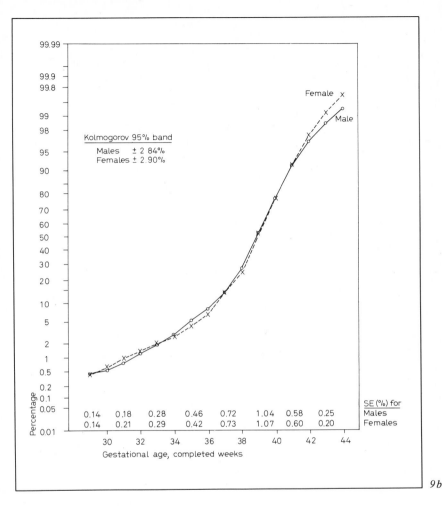

the reverse is usually the case. However, differences in that range are typically a lot smaller than two standard errors. Although the overall patterns for the two cities are by no means identical, they appear to be more similar than the corresponding patterns for birth weights. Percentage differences in the cumulatives for the three social class groups in Palermo are generally smaller than their birth weight counterparts. However, whilst there is a tendency for social class group 1 and 2 to show an aberrant pattern in the birth weight plots, social classes 4 and 5 tend to play this role in gestational age.

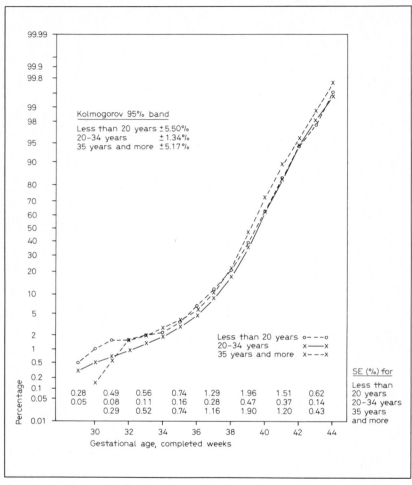

10a

Fig. 10. Cumulative distribution of gestational age of singletons by maternal age in Göteborg (a) and Palermo (b).

IV. Birth Length

Figure 12 shows that the cumulative distributions of birth length for singletons and twins follow the characteristic pattern for birth weights and gestational ages. We note that in the lower and middle parts of the range (where Palermo is quite ragged) there is little difference between the sample distributions for singletons, but that from 525 mm or so upwards, Palermo develops the characteristic heavy upper tail that we have seen previously for birth weight and gesta-

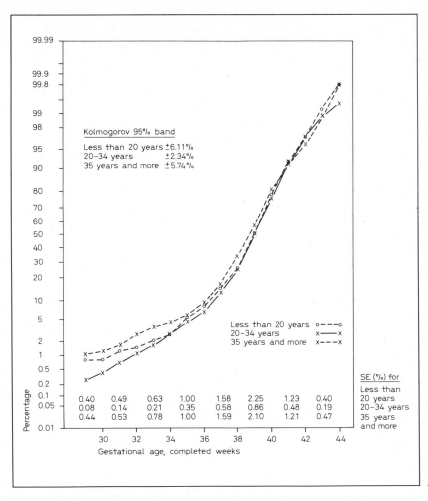

10b

tional age. So median lengths in the two cities appear to be similar and, if we take the data literally, we must conclude that it is Palermo rather than Göteborg which has the higher percentage of exceptionally long infants. However, table III shows that 6.4% lengths are unknown for Palermo even using the ESR sample. Since over one third of these are perinatal deaths, the sample curve almost certainly underestimates the true proportion in the lower tail. However, the distortion in the upper reaches is unlikely to be large. Certainly, the birth weight distribution of unknown birth lengths supports these contentions, as we shall see

Table III. Further details on cumulative distributions of birth length

Factor	Number (and percentage) of infants unclassified and their perinatal mortality rate	Sub-population within factor	Number of infants in sub-population (and percentage of total classified)	Number of infants of unknown birth length in sub-population	Percentage unknown in sub-population	Perinatal mortality rate for	
						total sub-population	infants of unknown birth length in sub-population
(a) Göteborg							
Multiplicity	none	singletons	12,039 (98.1)	25	0.2	11.4	320.0
	–	twins	232 (1.9)	1	0.4	86.2	1,000.0
		others	3 (0.0)	zero	zero	zero	zero
Sex	none	male	6,061 (50.3)	13	0.2	13.5	384.6
	–	female	5,978 (49.7)	12	0.2	9.2	250.0
Outcome	none	perinatal deaths	137 (1.1)	8	5.8	–	–
	–	survivors	11,902 (98.9)	17	0.1	–	–
Maternal age years	none	less than 20	653 (5.4)	1	0.2	13.8	zero
	–	20–34	10,669 (88.6)	21	0.2	10.7	285.7
		35 and more	717 (6.0)	3	0.4	19.5	666.7
Parity	none	parity 0	6,146 (51.1)	12	0.2	12.0	250.0
	–	1 and 2	5,282 (43.9)	12	0.2	8.7	333.3
		3 and more	611 (5.1)	1	0.2	27.8	1,000.0

(b) Palermo

Multiplicity*	none	singletons	4,656 (97.9)	300	6.4	32.0	356.7
	—	twins	93 (2.0)	26	28.0	107.5	115.4
		others	5 (0.1)	3	60.0	600.0	1,000.0
Sex*	1 (0.02)	male	2,374 (51.0)	162	6.8	33.7	358.0
	zero	female	2,281 (49.0)	138	6.0	30.3	355.1
Outcome*	none	perinatal deaths	149 (3.2)	107	71.8	—	—
	—	survivors	4,507 (96.8)	193	4.3	—	—
Maternal age* years	60 (1.3)	less than 20	520 (11.3)	33	6.3	28.8	333.3
	33.3	20–34	3,476 (75.6)	210	6.0	26.2	309.5
		35 and more	600 (13.1)	53	8.8	68.3	547.2
Parity*	36 (0.8)	parity 0	1,724 (37.3)	101	5.9	26.1	287.1
	83.3	1 and 2	1,998 (43.2)	97	4.9	22.0	319.6
		3 and more	898 (19.4)	96	10.7	63.5	458.3

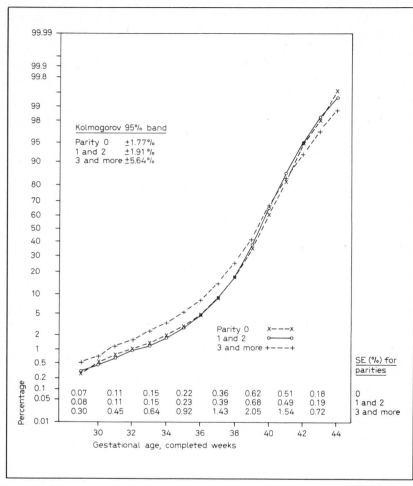

11a

Fig. 11. Cumulative distribution of gestational age of singletons by parity in Göteborg (a) and Palermo (b).

later on. Göteborg has 27 missing birth lengths out of 12,037 infants, seven of which are perinatal deaths. But although this will likely imply bias in the lower tail especially, the amount of distortion is likely to be small because of the small numbers involved. Later on, we shall see that about 50% of infants of unknown birth length have relatively low birth weights and that proportionately these are fairly well spread through the low birth weight range. Twins naturally show up as being shorter than singletons as well as lighter.

When the cumulatives are split by sex (fig. 13), we find that the sample

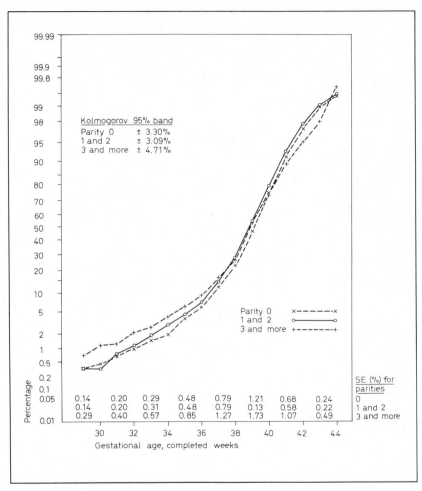

11b

curve for females almost always lies above that for males in both Göteborg and Palermo and usually significantly so. Although it appears from our data that males and females contain very similar proportions of low weight infants, the same cannot be said for birth length. At the sample median, males are about 3—4 mm longer at birth in Palermo and 6—7 mm in Göteborg.

Figure 14 displays birth length cumulatives broken down by the usual three maternal age groups, the plots for Palermo apparently being linear virtually nowhere. Qualitatively, these plots are similar to those for birth weight which is

what we might have anticipated, Palermo characteristically showing more variation in pattern. When the data are split by parity, however (fig. 15), Palermo
shows quite a different pattern from that for birth weight. Cumulatives are very
similar apart from in the upper parts of the range, where parity group 1 and 2
shows fewest infants proportionately. The same kind of behaviour is noticeable
for other than the lowest birth lengths in Göteborg. In particular, the considerable gap between parity 0 and 1 and 2 combined, which exists for birth weight,
is noticeably reduced in the upper parts of the range.

V. Head Circumference

Information on this indicator is available for Göteborg only and in principle
it has been measured to the nearest 5 mm; strong recorder preference (and
therefore bias) is shown for the multiples of 10 mm. So taken literally the
cumulative for our data will be an over-estimate at the 10s and underestimate at
the 5s. However, the general trend of the distribution is still apparent and we
show this in figure 16. In it, we have smoothed the cumulative by averaging
adjacent groups and this produces the typical mixture form for singletons that
Göteborg shows for the other three indicators. Since some 3% of head circumference measurements are unrecorded for singletons and more than 35% of these
are perinatal deaths, estimates of the distribution in the lower tail would be
unreliable even if recorder bias were not present.

VI. Joint Distributions of Measures of Maturity

Much more can be gained from studying the joint distribution of two
related variables and its parameters as a rule than from their separate univariate
distributions. For example, in our context knowing the joint distribution of
birth weight and gestational age allows us to follow the changes in the distribution of birth weight and related features as the level of gestational age is varied.
Knowledge of this relationship between the two characteristics can then be used
to judge whether any particular birth weight is an outlier given the associated
gestational age. Our three common indicators of maturity generate three pairs of
bivariate distributions and one that is trivariate. There is insufficient space here
to present details of all four, so we have confined our discussion to just two —
the joint distribution of birth weight and gestational age and that of birth weight
and birth length. In the case of Palermo, we have no option but to use the ESR
sample.

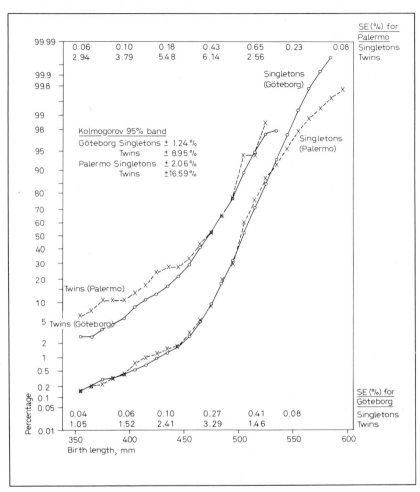

Fig. 12. Cumulative distribution of birth length by multiplicity of birth.

The distribution of most interest to paediatricians seems to be that of birth weight and gestational age and a basic summary of this for each city is given in table IV. Probably the most valuable single feature of the joint distribution is the conditional distribution of birth weight for given levels of gestational age and plots of this univariate distribution are set out in figure 17. Birth weight cumulatives for Göteborg are relatively linear for most gestational ages, indicating approximate single normal or Gaussian conditional distributions. However, the plot for 32 weeks and less suggests the presence of more than one normal

Table IV. Joint distribution of birth weight and gestational age

Birth weight, g	Gestational age, completed weeks											
	32 and less		33		34		35		36		37	
(a) Göteborg												
875 and less	15 (132)	(882) (1)	0		1 (15)	(59) (0)	0		0		0	
876–1,375	33 (289)	(660) (3)	6 (146)	(120) (0)	2 (31)	(40) (0)	0		4 (20)	(80) (0)	0	
1,376–1,875	31 (272)	(413) (3)	8 (195)	(107) (1)	8 (123)	(107) (1)	7 (59)	(93) (1)	5 (22)	(67) (0)	4 (9)	(53) (0)
1,876–2,375	16 (140)	(69) (1)	13 (317)	(56) (1)	20 (308)	(86) (2)	24 (203)	(103) (2)	23 (103)	(99) (2)	39 (86)	(168) (3)
2,376–2,875	14 (123)	(13) (1)	9 (220)	(9) (1)	20 (308)	(19) (2)	53 (449)	(50) (4)	77 (345)	(73) (6)	101 (222)	(96) (8)
2,876–3,375	3 (26)	(1) (0)	4 (98)	(1) (0)	8 (123)	(2) (1)	20 (169)	(5) (2)	75 (336)	(20) (6)	200 (440)	(54) (17)
3,376–3,875	2 (18)	(0) (0)	1 (24)	(0) (0)	5 (77)	(1) (0)	9 (76)	(2) (1)	34 (152)	(8) (3)	85 (187)	(19) (7)
3,876–4,375	0		0		1 (15)	(0) (0)	3 (25)	(1) (0)	5 (22)	(2) (0)	23 (51)	(11) (2)
4,376–4,875	0		0		0		2 (17)	(5) (0)	0		3 (7)	(8) (0)
4,876–5,375	0		0		0		0		0		0	
5,376 and more	0		0		0		0		0		0	
Unknown	0		0		0		0		0		0	
Total	114 (1,000)	(9) (9)	41 (1,000)	(3) (3)	65 (1,000)	(5) (5)	118 (1,000)	(10) (10)	223 (1,000)	(19) (19)	455 (1,000)	(38) (38)

component, so a working approximation for the joint distribution of birth weight and gestational age is likely to be a mixture of two or more bivariate normal distributions rather than a single. This conforms with the observation that both marginal distributions are mixed normal, and has appealing consistency.

	39		40		41		42 or more		unknown		total	
	0		0		0		0		1	(59)	17	(1,000)
									(2)	(0)	(1)	(1)
	1	(20)	0		0		0		4	(80)	50	(1,000)
	(0)	(0)							(9)	(0)	(4)	(4)
(80)	2	(27)	0		0		0		4	(53)	75	(1,000)
(0)	(1)	(0)							(9)	(0)	(6)	(6)
(56)	32	(138)	23	(99)	8	(34)	7	(30)	14	(60)	232	(1,000)
(1)	(15)	(3)	(7)	(2)	(3)	(1)	(4)	(1)	(30)	(1)	(19)	(19)
(160)	201	(190)	166	(157)	114	(108)	80	(76)	53	(50)	1,057	(1,000)
(14)	(91)	(17)	(54)	(14)	(48)	(9)	(41)	(7)	(113)	(4)	(88)	(88)
(105)	830	(224)	947	(255)	626	(169)	460	(124)	148	(40)	3,709	(1,000)
(32)	(377)	(69)	(309)	(79)	(262)	(52)	(238)	(38)	(317)	(12)	(308)	(308)
(66)	835	(189)	1,244	(282)	956	(217)	783	(177)	168	(38)	4,413	(1,000)
(24)	(379)	(69)	(405)	(103)	(400)	(79)	(405)	(65)	(360)	(14)	(367)	(367)
(39)	261	(128)	587	(287)	559	(273)	474	(232)	54	(26)	2,047	(1,000)
(7)	(119)	(22)	(191)	(49)	(234)	(46)	(245)	(39)	(116)	(4)	(170)	(170)
(28)	37	(95)	95	(243)	114	(292)	109	(279)	20	(51)	391	(1,000)
(1)	(17)	(3)	(31)	(8)	(48)	(9)	(56)	(9)	(43)	(2)	(32)	(32)
(43)	3	(65)	7	(152)	14	(304)	19	(413)	1	(22)	46	(1,000)
(0)	(1)	(0)	(2)	(1)	(6)	(1)	(10)	(2)	(2)	(0)	(4)	(4)
(500)	0		0		0		1	(500)	0		2	(1,000)
(0)							(1)	(0)			(0)	(0)
	0		0		0		0		0		0	
(80)	2,202	(183)	3,069	(255)	2,391	(199)	1,933	(161)	467	(39)	12,039	(1,000)
(80)	(1,000)	(183)	(1,000)	(255)	(1,000)	(199)	(1,000)	(161)	(1,000)	(39)	(1,000)	(1,000)

The Palermo data on the other hand are less linear with the characteristic long upper tail evident for most gestational ages. It is instructive to superimpose one set of plots on the other. What we find among the lower gestational ages is that the plot for Palermo lies entirely to the right of that for Göteborg, the gap being considerable. This indicates a sizeable difference in birth weight for a given

Table IV (continued)

Birth weight, g	Gestational age, completed weeks										
	32 and less		33		34		35		36		37
(b) Palermo											
875 and less	6 (750)	1 (125)	0		0		0		0		
	(103) (1)	(38) (0)									
876–1,375	11 (688)	0		0		1 (63)	0		1 (63)		
	(190) (2)					(12) (0)			(4) (0)		
1,376–1,875	16 (500)	4 (125)	4 (125)		1 (31)	1 (31)	2 (63)				
	(276) (3)	(154) (1)	(95) (1)		(12) (0)	(8) (0)	(7) (0)				
1,876–2,375	(10) (119)	9 (107)	11 (131)		8 (95)	7 (83)	8 (95)				
	(172) (2)	(346) (2)	(262) (2)		(96) (2)	(58) (2)	(28) (2)				
2,376–2,875	8 (25)	5 (16)	12 (38)		24 (75)	27 (85)	48 (150)				
	(138) (2)	(192) (1)	(286) (3)		(293) (5)	(225) (6)	(168) (10)				
2,876–3,375	3 (3)	3 (3)	11 (10)		22 (20)	50 (45)	100 (90)				
	(52) (1)	(115) (1)	(262) (2)		(268) (5)	(417) (11)	(351) (21)				
3,376–3,875	2 (1)	3 (2)	2 (1)		15 (9)	17 (10)	89 (51)				
	(34) (0)	(115) (1)	(48) (0)		(183) (3)	(142) (4)	(312) (19)				
3,876–4,375	1 (1)	1 (1)	2 (2)		6 (7)	11 (12)	25 (28)				
	(17) (0)	(38) (0)	(48) (0)		(73) (1)	(92) (2)	(88) (5)				
4,376–4,875	0	0	0		3 (11)	4 (15)	6 (22)				
					(37) (1)	(33) (1)	(21) (1)				
4,876–5,375	0	0	0		0	1 (17)	1 (17)				
						(8) (0)	(4) (0)				
5,376 and more	0	0	0		0	0	1 (59)				
							(4) (0)				
Unknown	1 (9)	0	0		2 (18)	2 (18)	4 (35)				
	(17) (0)				(24) (0)	(17) (0)	(14) (1)				
Total	58 (12)	26 (6)	42 (9)		82 (16)	120 (26)	285 (61)				
	(1,000) (12)	(1,000) (6)	(1,000) (9)		(1,000) (16)	(1,000) (26)	(1,000) (61)				

gestational age if this age is relatively low. However, the gap between the two narrows appreciably among the higher gestational ages. This pattern is not too surprising, considering that average birth weight for Palermo and Göteborg is similar overall and that average gestational age for Palermo is definitely lower than that for Göteborg. So amalgamation of all 'light for dates' infants, for

		39		40		41		42 or more		unknown		total	
		0		0		0		0		1 (125) (6) (0)		8 (1,000) (2) (2)	
		0		0		0		0		3 (188) (18) (1)		16 (1,000) (3) (3)	
(31) (0)		0		1 (31) (1) (0)		0		1 (31) (3) (0)		1 (31) (6) (0)		32 (1,000) (7) (7)	
(60) (1)		11 (131) (10) (2)		5 (60) (4) (1)		2 (24) (3) (0)		1 (12) (3) (0)		7 (83) (42) (2)		84 (1,000) (18) (18)	
(135) (9)		56 (176) (49) (12)		41 (129) (37) (9)		21 (66) (31) (5)		19 (60) (50) (4)		15 (47) (89) (3)		319 (1,000) (69) (69)	
(161) 5) (38)		281 (254) (245) (60)		221 (200) (197) (47)		118 (107) (173) (25)		79 (71) (208) (17)		41 (37) (244) (9)		1,107 (1,000) (238) (238)	
(122) 5) (45)		454 (263) (395) (98)		479 (277) (428) (103)		265 (153) (389) (57)		137 (79) (361) (29)		55 (32) (327) (12)		1,729 (1,000) (371) (371)	
(69) 3) (13)		237 (265) (206) (51)		246 (275) (220) (53)		192 (214) (282) (41)		90 (100) (237) (19)		23 (26) (137) (5)		896 (1,000) (192) (192)	
(88) ·) (5)		62 (226) (54) (13)		73 (266) (65) (16)		62 (226) (91) (13)		30 (109) (79) (6)		10 (36) (60) (2)		274 (1,000) (59) (59)	
(50) ») (1)		10 (167) (9) (2)		18 (300) (16) (4)		13 (217) (19) (3)		12 (200) (32) (3)		2 (33) (12) (0)		60 (1,000) (13) (13)	
(59) (0)		6 (353) (5) (1)		4 (235) (4) (1)		1 (59) (1) (0)		4 (235) (11) (1)		0		17 (1,000) (4) (4)	
(175) ») (4)		31 (272) (27) (7)		31 (272) (28) (7)		7 (61) (10) (2)		6 (53) (16) (1)		10 (88) (60) (2)		114 (1,000) (24) (24)	
3 (118) 000) (118)		1,148 (247) (1,000) (118)		1,119 (240) (1,000) (247)		681 (146) (1,000) (240)		379 (81) (1,000) (146)		168 (36) (1,000) (81)		4,656 (1,000) (1,000) (36)	

example, would be misleading, since relative behaviour in the two cities is strongly age-dependent. In figure 18, we have plotted out the 10, 50 and 90% sample points of these conditional distributions, and these naturally also show this narrowing effect from 35 weeks onwards. The median weight for Palermo at 35 weeks exceeds that of Göteborg by some 350 g, but this has been reduced to

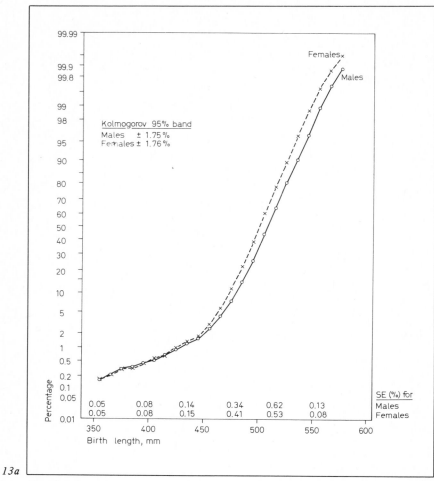

13a

Fig. 13. Cumulative distribution of birth length of singletons by sex in Göteborg (a) and Palermo (b).

150 g by 40 weeks. The 90% points show much less convergence due to the characteristic heavy upper tail of Palermo. The comparison between the two cities is obviously complicated by the fact that the natural gestational ages to delivery are different, and it may be that we should replace gestational age by gestational age/average gestational age or something similar. This certainly has the effect of bringing the conditional distributions more into line. As they stand in uncorrected form, the differences are so large that the application of either in the other city could be very misleading. These conclusions are of course based

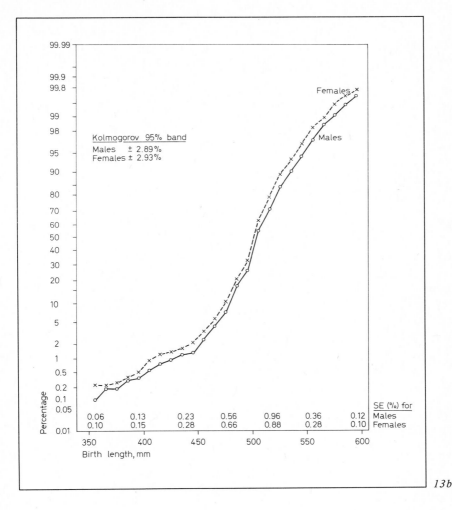

13b

on the infants whose birth weight and gestational age are recorded. However, missing percentages in both cities could affect the conclusions. In particular, we might note that highest percentages of unknown gestational ages for Palermo tend to occur among the lowest birth weights (total of 8.6% for infants of weight less than 2,375 g, for example) whereas those for Göteborg in relative percentages tend to be more evenly spread.

At present, paediatricians commonly use sample percentage points of these distributions. However, given that sample sizes are not too large, we are con-

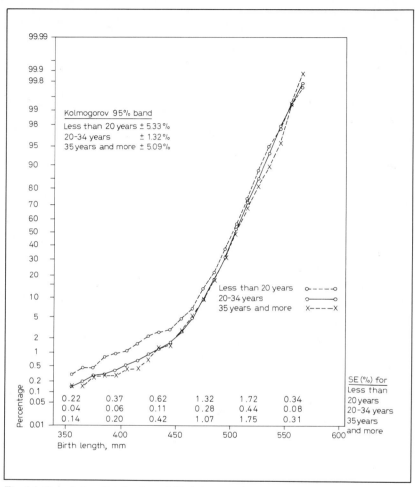

14a

Fig. 14. Cumulative distribution of birth length of singletons by maternal age in Göteborg (a) and Palermo (b).

vinced that model building here will repay the effort, and one of us (R.A.H.) is currently working on the problem. It is worth pointing out that it is only through using models that all of the observations can be used efficiently to estimate each percentage point. In the case of Göteborg, at all except the lowest gestational ages the birth weight distribution can be approximated by a single normal distribution for which the mean and median coincide. Neither of these things is true for the lowest gestational ages, and it is not clear to us whether the median regression curve is more valuable than the mean regression curve in this

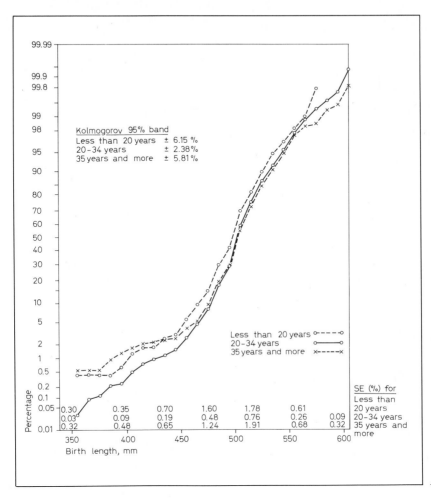

14b

case. What is incontrovertible is that both are non-linear. A further point to bear in mind is that if the mixture model really is appropriate for the joint distribution (and it seems very likely), then we must recognize that there are two quite different regression or growth curves, rather than just one.

Looking at this distribution's natural partner, the conditional distribution of gestational age given birth weight, we find what we might have anticipated. Palermo shows considerably lower average gestational age for a given birth weight, the whole distribution being clearly displaced to the left in comparison

Table V. Joint distribution of birth weight and birth length

Birth weight, g	Birth length, mm				
	355 and less	365–385	386–415	416–445	446–475
(a) Göteborg					
875 and less	13 (765) (722) (1)	2 (118) (87) (0)	1 (59) (24) (0)	0	0
876–1,375	5 (100) (278) (0)	19 (380) (826) (2)	18 (360) (439) (1)	4 (80) (34) (0)	2 (40) (2) (0)
1,376–1,875	0	1 (13) (43) (0)	21 (280) (512) (2)	42 (560) (362) (3)	9 (120) (10) (1)
1,876–2,375	0	0	1 (4) (24) (0)	55 (237) (474) (5)	142 (612) (152) (12)
2,376–2,875	0	1 (1) (43) (0)	0	15 (14) (129) (1)	486 (460) (521) (40)
2,876–3,375	0	0	0	0	284 (77) (304) (24)
3,376–3,875	0	0	0	0	10 (2) (11) (1)
3,876–4,375	0	0	0	0	0
4,376–4,875	0	0	0	0	0
4,876–5,375	0	0	0	0	0
5,376 and more	0	0	0	0	0
Unknown	0	0	0	0	0
Total	18 (1) (1,000) (1)	23 (2) (1,000) (2)	41 (3) (1,000) (3)	116 (10) (1,000) (10)	933 (77) (1,000) (77)

with Göteborg. For this distribution, there is a much smaller tendency for the differential between the two cities to narrow as we increase the fixed birth weight level, which is not surprising since average gestational age is lower in Palermo.

Moving now to the joint distribution of birth weight and birth length, we

-505	506–535	536–565	566-595	596 and more	unknown	total
	0	0	0	0	1 (59)	17 (1,000)
					(40) (0)	(1) (1)
	0	0	0	0	2 (40)	50 (1,000)
					(80) (0)	(4) (4)
	0	0	0	0	2 (27)	75 (1,000)
					(80) (0)	(6) (6)
(121)	1 (4)	0	0	0	5 (22)	232 (1,000)
(2)	(0) (0)				(200) (0)	(19) (19)
(500)	21 (20)	0	0	0	5 (5)	1,057 (1,000)
) (44)	(4) (2)				(200) (0)	(88) (88)
9 (741)	662 (178)	8 (2)	0	0	6 (2)	3,709 (1,000)
) (228)	(134) (55)	(10) (1)			(240) (0)	(308) (308)
8 (373)	2,601 (589)	151 (34)	2 (0)	0	1 (0)	4,413 (1,000)
) (137)	(528) (216)	(189) (13)	(74) (0)		(40) (0)	(367) (367)
(83)	1,467 (717)	401 (196)	7 (3)	0	3 (1)	2,047 (1,000)
(12)	(298) (122)	(501) (33)	(259) (1)		(120) (0)	(170) (170)
(3)	168 (430)	212 (542)	9 (23)	1 (3)	0	391 (1,000)
(0)	(34) (14)	(265) (18)	(333) (1)	(500) (0)		(32) (32)
	10 (217)	28 (609)	7 (152)	1 (22)	0	46 (1,000)
	(2) (1)	(35) (2)	(259) (1)	(500) (0)		(4) (4)
	0	0	2 (1,000)	0	0	2 (1,000)
			(74) (0)			(0) (0)
	0	0	0	0	0	0
4 (426)	4,930 (410)	800 (66)	27 (2)	2 (0)	25 (2)	12,039 (1,000)
00) (426)	(1,000) (410)	(1,000) (66)	(1,000) (2)	(1,000) (0)	(1,000) (2)	(1,000) (1,000)

find this summarized in table V for the two cities. Again, a study of the distributions of birth weight for fixed values of birth length (fig. 19) is instructive. Göteborg shows almost linear cumulatives among the higher length groups, but interference from a secondary component in the joint distribution is evident from the plot for 475 mm or less. In some ways, Palermo is similar, but the

Table V (continued)

Birth weight, g	Birth length, mm									
	355 and less		365–385		386–415		416–445		446–475	
(b) Palermo										
875 and less	2 (286)	(250) (0)	0		0		0		0	
876–1,375	3 (429)	(188) (1)	2 (250)	(125) (0)	0		0		0	
1,376–1,875	0		4 (500)	(125) (1)	10 (345)	(312) (2)	3 (91)	(94) (1)	1 (3)	(31) (0)
1,876–2,375	0		0		9 (310)	(107) (2)	13 (394)	(155) (3)	20 (64)	(238) (4)
2,376–2,875	1 (143)	(3) (0)	0		3 (103)	(9) (1)	8 (242)	(25) (2)	87 (278)	(273) (19)
2,876–3,375	1 (143)	(1) (0)	1 (125)	(1) (0)	3 (103)	(3) (1)	5 (152)	(5) (1)	103 (329)	(93) (22)
3,376–3,875	0		1 (125)	(1) (0)	2 (69)	(1) (0)	2 (61)	(1) (0)	75 (240)	(43) (16)
3,876–4,375	0		0		1 (34)	(1) (0)	1 (30)	(1) (0)	13 (42)	(15) (3)
4,376–4,875	0		0		0		0		4 (13)	(15) (1)
4,876–5,375	0		0		0		0		1 (3)	(17) (0)
5,376 and more	0		0		0		0		0	
Unknown	0		0		1 (34)	(9) (0)	1 (30)	(9) (0)	9 (29)	(79) (2)
Total	7 (1,000)	(2) (2)	8 (1,000)	(2) (2)	29 (1,000)	(6) (6)	33 (1,000)	(7) (7)	313 (1,000)	(67) (67)

characteristic heavy upper tail is present for almost all birth lengths and therefore single Gaussian distributions are not appropriate. Superimposing the plots for Göteborg on those for Palermo, we note first that for any given birth length the slope of the Göteborg cumulative is noticeably larger than that of Palermo, indicating less variation in Göteborg, and that the Palermo curves show a much

–505	506–535	536–565	566-595	596 and more	unknown	total
	0	0	0	0	6 (750) (20) (1)	8 (1,000) (2) (2)
	0	0	0	0	11 (688) (37) (2)	16 (1,000) (3) (3)
(31) (0)	0	0	0	0	13 (406) (43) (3)	32 (1,000) (7) (7)
(107) (2)	0	0	0	0	33 (393) (110) (7)	84 (1,000) (18) (18)
(505) (35)	17 (53) (12) (4)	3 (9) (10) (1)	0	0	39 (122) (130) (8)	319 (1,000) (69) (69)
(639) (152)	201 (182) (142) (43)	26 (23) (87) (6)	2 (2) (47) (0)	1 (1) (83) (0)	57 (51) (190) (12)	1,107 (1,000) (238) (238)
(513) (191)	601 (348) (424) (129)	83 (48) (278) (18)	8 (5) (186) (2)	0	70 (40) (233) (15)	1,729 (1,000) (371) (371)
(347) (67)	414 (462) (292) (89)	99 (110) (331) (21)	20 (22) (465) (4)	4 (4) (333) (1)	33 (37) (110) (7)	896 (1,000) (192) (192)
(234) (14)	120 (438) (85) (26)	62 (226) (207) (13)	5 (18) (116) (1)	3 (11) (250) (1)	16 (58) (53) (3)	274 (1,000) (59) (59)
(150) (2)	19 (317) (13) (4)	18 (300) (60) (4)	4 (67) (93) (1)	2 (33) (167) (0)	7 (117) (23) (2)	60 (1,000) (13) (13)
(59) (0)	4 (235) (3) (1)	4 (235) (13) (1)	3 (176) (68) (1)	2 (118) (167) (0)	3 (176) (10) (1)	17 (1,000) (4) (4)
(377) (9)	43 (377) (30) (9)	4 (35) (13) (1)	1 (9) (23) (0)	0	12 (105) (40) (3)	114 (1,000) (24) (24)
03 (471) 00) (471)	1,419 (305) (1,000) (305)	299 (64) (1,000) (64)	43 (9) (1,000) (9)	12 (3) (1,000) (3)	300 (64) (1,000) (64)	4,656 (1,000) (1,000) (1,000)

stronger bunching effect. For the shortest infants, the cumulative for Göteborg lies entirely to the left of that for Palermo, indicating higher birth weight in Palermo for a given length. However (as with gestational age), this discrepancy narrows as birth length is increased and by the time we reach 506—535 mm the two curves intersect (strongly). The same behaviour is also illustrated in fig-

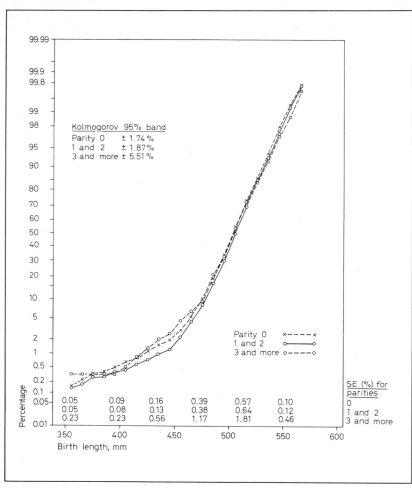

15a

Fig. 15. Cumulative distribution of birth length of singletons by parity in Göteborg (a) and Palermo (b).

ure 20, where we have again plotted out sample percentage points of the distributions. By the highest lengths, it is Göteborg which is showing the higher 10 and 50% points, though because of the long upper tail of Palermo, the two 90% points just about coincide. So any comparison involving a function of the two measures like grams weight per millimetre of length has to be made at each level of birth length, or is otherwise misleading. In terms of the average or median, if we take the data literally, we have to conclude that short infants weigh considerably more in Palermo, whilst long infants weigh heavier in Göteborg

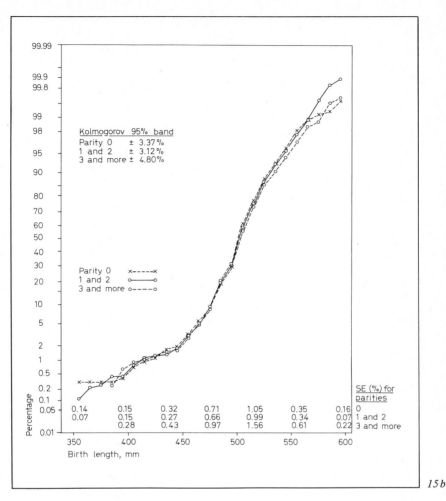

15b

(though a higher percentage of very long infants are very heavy in Palermo). So the fact that both average birth weight and birth length are very similar for the two cities conceals very considerable differences in pattern between them. Again all of these conclusions refer to infants whose measurements were recorded. However, for some low birth weight groups in Palermo percentages of unknown birth lengths must be noted (45% of the lengths of infants weighing less than 2,375 g are unknown, for example), and this could easily affect our conclusions.

Comparing instead the conditional distributions of birth length for given

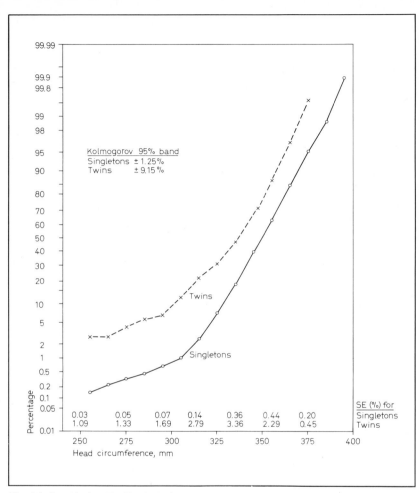

Fig. 16. Cumulative distribution of head circumference for Göteborg.

birth weight, we find an even wider difference in slope of the two cumulatives, Göteborg again showing less variation for a given birth weight. The overall pattern in the two sets of conditional curves is quite similar to that seen previously for birth weight given birth length. However, the curves begin to intersect at relatively much lower levels of the conditioning variable. Göteborg again shows a clear pattern with well-spaced and (almost) single Gaussian curves for the higher weights. By comparison the bunching tendency in Palermo is very noticeable and almost all of its conditional cumulatives are S-shaped even on the probit scale.

VII. Conclusions and Comment

In this section of the monograph, we have compared the distributions of some maturity indicators and their parameters for the two cities. Indicators studied singly are birth weight, gestational age, birth length and, for Göteborg only, head circumference. We have also looked at the joint distributions of birth weight and gestational age and birth weight and birth length.

Birth weights are measured to the nearest 10 g in our surveys in principle, but in practice we find that recorders have favoured attractively rounded numbers like 2,000 and 2,500 g. This 'digit preference' shows up much more strongly in the Palermo survey than the Göteborg and must not be overlooked when studying distributions. If 2,500 g were to be used as an end-point of a birth weight group, then clearly at that point the sample cumulative plot would be a strongly upward biased estimate. Much birth weight data is reported regrettably in this form. We can avoid this undesirable bias to some extent by choosing less conventional boundary points like 2,625 g and these are used throughout this paper.

There is little doubt that median birth weights over all singletons are similar in Göteborg and Palermo, but that Göteborg shows less variation. More surprising, perhaps, is the fact that the proportions of low weight infants *appear to be* almost identical (fig. 1). However, although the coverage of birth weight in Palermo is very high (95%) compared with most surveys, the missing 5% could easily upset the low weight pattern observed. Observed proportions of infants weighing 2,500 g or less amount to some 5% also, so if all the missing birth weights in Palermo were low, then Palermo would be showing a rate double that of Göteborg. This is extremely unlikely of course, but the perinatal mortality rate of the missing 5% is identical to the birth weight specific mortality rate for infants of 2,500 g or so in Palermo, and in view of this and other things the true low birth rate in Palermo could easily be 25–50% higher than that in Göteborg. The probable effect of missing observations on the birth weight distribution and its parameters should *always* be assessed in some way or another, but is often completely ignored in perinatal surveys. The apparent similarity of the two cumulative distributions is not matched in the highest weights. The Palermo curve shows a very long upper tail, indicating a much higher percentage of very heavy infants. Possible reasons for this include the inhomogeneity of the population and variations in diet, but more information would be need to resolve this question. Partly because of the behaviour in the high weights, but not completely, a mathematical model (mixture of Gaussian distributions) that we have used hitherto to summarize birth weight distributions in the US and UK does not appear to fit the Palermo data adequately. However, this is not true of the Göteborg data, which fit the 'mixture' pattern well. On splitting singletons by either the age of mother or parity, we find clear differences in the distributional pattern of birth weight between the two cities. Doubtless, some of this is due to

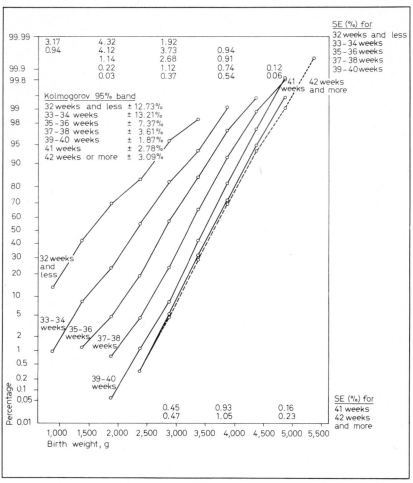

17a

Fig. 17. Cumulative distribution of birth weight for fixed levels of gestational age in Göteborg (a) and Palermo (b).

differences in the distributions of maternal ages and parity over the two cities, but it seems very likely that other (and hitherto unidentified) factors are also making their presence felt.

The shapes of the distributions of gestational age over all singletons for the two cities appear to be similar to their birth weight counterparts, Palermo again showing a long upper tail (fig. 8). However, their relative locations are quite different, with Palermo singletons seemingly some 4—5 days younger on average at delivery. Some difference in this direction was expected, but its extent com-

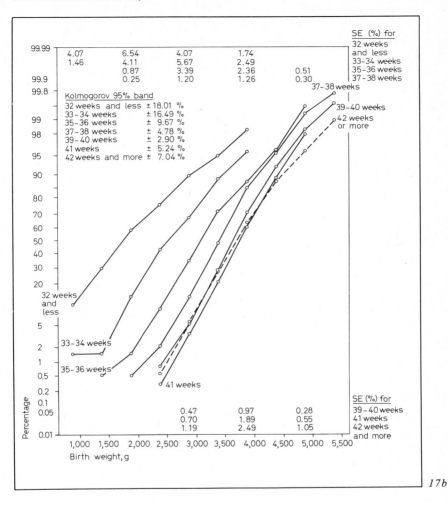

17b

plicates the comparison of the joint distributions of birth weight and gestational age upon which we comment later. The missing gestational ages in both cities (as well as undetected errors) could reduce this difference in medians but seem more likely to increase it. There is a very clear difference in the pattern between the two cities when the gestational ages of singletons are split by sex. In Göteborg, we see a higher percentage of males than females with low gestational age (the difference actually extending up to 40 weeks or so), whilst in Palermo the two distributions are very similar. The pattern for Palermo is unusual and unex-

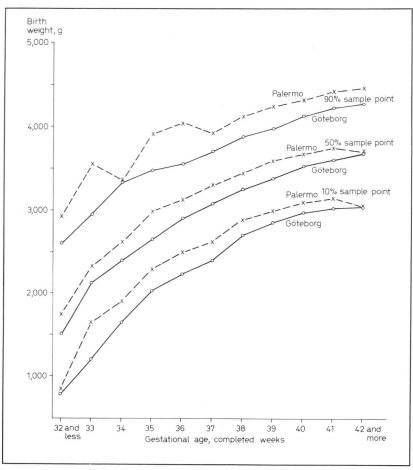

Fig. 18. Some percentage points of the distribution of birth weight at various gestational ages.

plained. Differences also exist in the distributional patterns for the two cities when the data are split by maternal age. For either city, the distributional patterns for gestational age and birth weight after splitting by maternal age or parity are also quite different.

Our third maturity indicator, birth length, adds to the consistency of the overall pattern since cumulative distributions for this over all singletons are similar in shape to those for both birth weight and gestational age in each city, just as we might expect (fig. 12). We find, in addition, that the distributional pattern for birth length in the two cities is much closer to that for birth weight than gestational age, which is not surprising either. Taking the data literally, the median birth lengths for the two cities are almost identical. Proportions of very short infants appear to be very similar too. However, since the 6.4% missing birth lengths for Palermo have a perinatal mortality rate ten times that of the ESR sample as a whole, it is very likely that the proportion of infants of short length at Palermo is significantly higher than it is in Göteborg (just as it is for birth weight). When the plots are broken down by maternal age, each city follows a similar pattern to the one shown for birth weight, but this is by no means true for the parity sub-populations. Although proportions of low weight males and females seem to be very similar in each city, the same is not true for birth length. In this case, percentages of short length females are some 40% higher than males at the 5th percentiles of the distributions for males.

Head circumference was recorded in Göteborg only and in principle measured to the nearest 5 mm. However, there is evidence in the data of much stronger recorder preference for the 10 mm points than the 5 mm. (Much of the bias would here be eliminated if it was in fact measured to the nearest 10 mm instead.) Even so, after smoothing, the distribution of head circumference conforms closely in shape to those of the other three indicators that we have studied, so lending even more weight to the 'mixture' hypothesis originally put forward by *Brimblecombe et al.* (1968).

From the joint distribution of birth weight and gestational age, we have derived the conditional distribution of birth weight for given levels of gestational age. A study of these distributions shows the regression or 'growth' curves in the two cities to be very different. Median birth weight in Palermo is much higher than in Göteborg among the low gestational ages, but this gap has narrowed considerably by 40 weeks or so. This pattern is not too surprising since median gestational age is definitely lower in Palermo overall, whilst average birth weight is about the same. The difference between the two growth curves is noticeably reduced if we replace gestational age by the ratio of gestational age/median gestational age. However, combining growth curve data from different sources to produce a single standard is potentially misleading, even if a suitable transformation of gestational age is used. A further point worth noting from these conditional distributions is that Palermo shows a long upper tail at *all* levels of gestational age, indicating that this feature is very firmly embedded in the data indeed. Even though many of the corresponding Göteborg plots are almost linear, so indicating single normal distributions approximately, the data as a whole strongly suggest that the joint distribution of birth weight and gestational age contains more than one bivariate normal component. If this is the case, perhaps we ought to be thinking in terms of two or more distinct growth curves rather than combining them to form just one. We are currently in the process of resolving the overall mixture into its component parts and intend to report on our findings when they become firm.

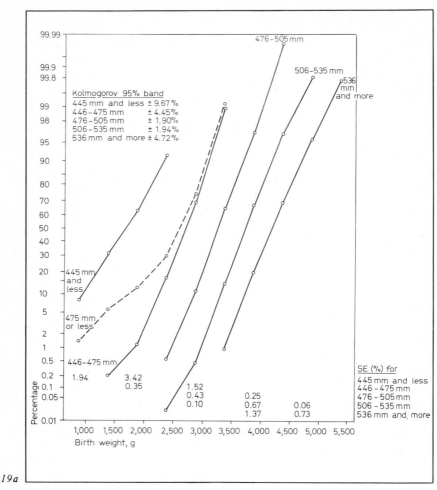

Fig. 19. Cumulative distribution of birth weight for fixed levels of birth length in Göteborg (a) and Palermo (b).

A study of the birth weight distributions at fixed levels of birth length shows that very considerable differences in pattern exist between the two cities, even though their average birth weights and lengths are similar. Our data appear to show that on average short infants weight more in Palermo whilst long infants weigh more in Göteborg. Hence, any attempt to compare 'shape' (assuming it to be some function of birth weight and length) would be very misleading unless carried out at fixed levels of length or weight, just as any comparison of 'light for dates' infants between the two cities would have to be carried out at fixed

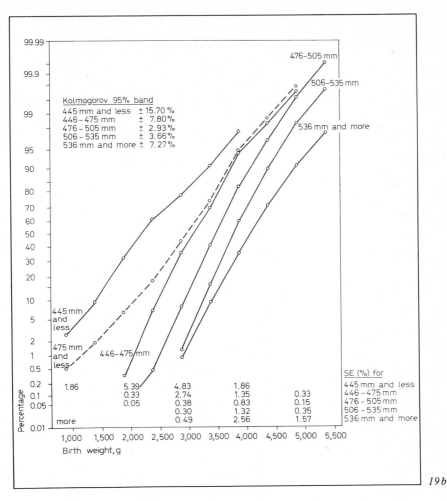

19b

levels of gestational age (or some function of it) to be relevant. These conclusions ought to be regarded as tentative rather than firm, since missing proportions in these joint distributions are occasionally high for Palermo.

Summary

In this paper, we present a simple descriptive statistical analysis of some well-accepted indicators of maturity, namely birth weight, gestational age and

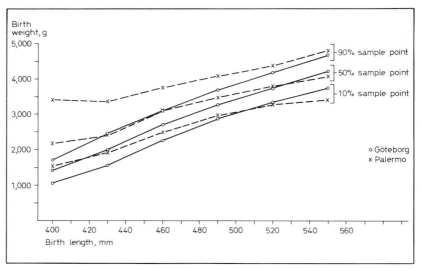

Fig. 20. Some percentage points of the distribution of birth weight for various levels of birth length.

birth length for the two cities. For Göteborg only, we also look briefly at head circumference. These are studied in some detail singly and to a lesser extent jointly. There seems to be little doubt that median birth weight and birth length in the two cities are similar and that Göteborg generally shows rather less variability. This difference in variation is largely due to the fact that the Palermo distributions have much longer upper tails. Such behaviour is quite untypical of the birth weight distributions from the US and UK that we have seen previously, and prevents an adequate fit of a mathematical model that we have successfully used hitherto to summarize birth weight data, namely a mixture of Gaussian distributions. Göteborg, on the other hand, conforms closely to UK patterns. Proportions of both low weight and short length infants appear to be very comparable in the two cities, but the nature and extent of missing observations from Palermo strongly suggest that our raw data underestimates the true proportions in that city. Cumulative plots for gestational age have the same general shape as those for birth weight and length, so producing a satisfying consistency. However, there is little doubt that infants in Palermo have a gestational age at least 4–5 days lower on average than those from Göteborg.

Growth curves (plots of median birth weight by gestational age) appear to be quite different in the two cities. Infants of low gestational age tend to weigh considerably more in Palermo, but this excess is largely eliminated by the time 40 weeks is reached. The contrast between the distributions of birth weight for fixed levels of birth length is stronger still, since on average short infants weigh more in Palermo, whilst long infants weigh more in Göteborg. However, missing percentages of observations for these conditional distributions are sometimes large for Palermo and so our conclusions should be considered tentative rather than firm.

Reference

Brimblecombe, F.S.W.; Ashford, J.R., and Fryer, J.G.: Significance of low birth weight in perinatal mortality. Br. J. prev. Soc. Med. *22:* 27–35 (1968).

Prof. *J. Fryer,* Department of Mathematical Statistics and Operational Research, University of Exeter, Streatham Court, Rennes Drive, *Exeter EX4 4PU* (England)

Section IV

Monogr. Paediat., vol. 9, pp. 86–120 (Karger, Basel 1977)

Clinical Analyses of Causes of Death with Emphasis on Perinatal Mortality[1]

P. Karlberg, A. Priolisi, T. Landström and U. Selstam

Department of Pediatrics, University of Göteborg, Göteborg and Child Health Institute, University of Palermo, Palermo

Background

The human spends the first one-fourth of life in growth and development preparing for the remainder of life. The first one-hundredth part of expected life is spent *in utero* as a highly sheltered existence, and is the biologically most intensive period of an individual's development. After the prenatal period, the human has all its organs and most functions developed or under development.

Birth, the transfer from a sheltered intrauterine existence to an extrauterine existence requiring a functionally independent individual, involves, by definition, a dramatic adaptation of practically all body functions during the neonatal period. The most critical adaptations are related to the transfer of gaseous exchange with the surrounding atmosphere, from transplacental exchange via the mother, to transpulmonary exchange via the newborn infant's lungs (*Smith and Nelson,* 1976). There is also an immediately increased demand on energy metabolism, mainly for maintenance of homeostasis and of body temperature at the increased heat loss from the body surface. The energy supply has now to be met by nutrition, digestion and absorption. The intensity of a series of control mechanisms will increase. All new sensory impulses have to be processed, learned, appreciated, and organized for future development.

In the normal full-term fetus/newborn infant, the entire process seems to occur through pregnancy, delivery and neonatal adaptation without any apparent specific effort. However, the development from conception to the state of a functionally independent newborn infant involves a series of interrelated events. Interferences are not unusual, sometimes causing disturbances of a transient character, sometimes resulting in irreversible damage with late sequelae or, in extreme cases, in perinatal death.

[1] The Göteborg study is supported by a grant from The Bank of Sweden Tercentenary Foundation.

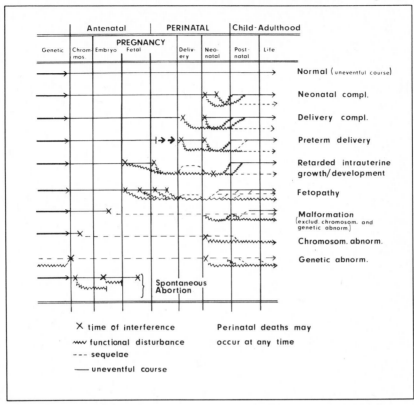

Fig. 1. Relation of time of original interference, and time of functional significance. The neonatal period – the 'show-up' time.

Thus, the *outcome* may vary within a wide spectrum: (1) From fetal death before 28 completed weeks of gestation – a spontaneous abortion. (2) Late fetal death after 28 completed weeks, before or during delivery – a stillbirth. (3) Neonatal death, death during the functional adaptive period after birth, early neonatal death within the first 7 days; late neonatal death between 7 and 28 days. (4) Passage through the perinatal period with irreversible damage of antenatal or perinatal origin: (a) with severe damage, the sequelae are already apparent in the neonatal period; (b) with medium damage, first apparent during infancy; (c) with slight damage, however, the sequelae may be difficult to recognize even in later childhood and adolescence. (5) To intact survival.

The graph in figure 1 illustrates some of the main possibilities in relation to time of the original interference and time of functional significance, emphasizing the neonatal period as the 'show-up' time. Delivery in itself means mechanical

Table I. Number of stillbirths, early neonatal deaths, late neonatal deaths, and late infant deaths in relation to place of delivery

Place of delivery	Total number of births	Stillbirths	Early neonatal deaths (up to 7 days)	Late neonatal deaths (from 7 up to 28 days)	Late infant deaths (from 28 days up to 1 year)	Total number of deaths
Göteborg						
West Hospital	5,585	48	34	5	5	92
East Hospital	6,686	31	44	3	20	98
Total	12,271	79	78	8	25	190
Palermo						
University Hospital	1,099	36	23	14	1	74
Hospital A	1,708	86	57	48	11	202
Hospital B	1,386	46	31	24	5	106
Hospital A or B	634	29	7	2		38
Private clinic	4,994	40	37	32	12	121
Home	3,232	35	23	22	17	97
Unknown	135	5	20	9	2	36
Total	13,188	277	198	151	48	674

and, above all, functional strain. A mis-timed event, such as a preterm delivery, may mean that the birth itself will exert a great strain on a vulnerable immature individual and/or the functional adaptation after birth may be an overwhelming strain on the unprepared immature fetus. Retarded growth and development prenatally may also lead to a vulnerable state, though of another kind. Feto-pathies caused by prenatal infections (TORCH), isoimmunization (Rh), meta-bolic disorders (for example, maternal diabetes) may induce a vulnerable state, but also severe clinical conditions by themselves. Malformations caused by disturbances in the first trimester will usually have functional consequences that begin during neonatal adaptation, as is also the case with chromosomal and genetic abnormalities if not ended by an early spontaneous abortion.

Clearly, the period around birth has great biomedical impact; critical func-tional changes occur that are at risk from so many factors. The actual outcome depends on the degree of any disturbance and the relation between the distur-bance and the ability of the fetus/newborn infant to counteract such.

Although intact survival is the dominant outcome in all populations, deaths and irreversible damage are obviously of great importance. Not only because of their proportions (3−10% of all newborn babies), but also because they repre-sent one extreme of the spectrum of varying outcomes due to the interplay between different factors. Thus, the analysis of the underlying mechanisms involved will have a broader meaning than for just deaths before 28 days of postnatal life, allowing evaluation of the effect of preventive and therapeutic measures and for the rational utilization of available resources for perinatal care.

Aim

This section deals with a clinical analysis of the *functional cause of perinatal death and late neonatal death* in order to identify areas of priority within pre-ventive and curative care. Death during later infancy is also included. The meth-odology used in this analysis can also be utilized as an appropriate short-time tool in clinical practice to focus on the principal problems encountered leading to more useful multidisciplinary efforts for the improvement of perinatal and infant care.

Material

The stillbirths and deaths during infancy in the Göteborg and Palermo surveys, de-scribed in section I, form the material for this analysis. In the two total birth populations of 12,271 and 13,188, respectively, there were 190 and 674 deaths. The groupings in terms of vital statistics as well as the distribution of the different places of delivery are shown in table I.

Method of Analyses

1) Analysis of information on (a) condition on death evaluated from clinical assessment and, when available, postmortem examination; (b) the course of events/disorders/diseases in relation to the physical characteristics of the newborn infant at birth, and the expected functional adaptation to extrauterine life in the event of live birth.

2) A main functional cause of death (FCD) determined for each individual case.

3) Evaluation of growth and development, and maturity, at birth.

Main Functional Groups

a) First trimester or earlier disturbances: gametopathy, embryopathy, signficant malformations, heart malformations.

b) Second/third trimester disturbances: fetopathy (example: Rh-isoimmunization/hydrops and prenatal infection [TORCH]).

c) Traumatic brain lesion due to complication during delivery (example: tentorial rupture with hemorrhage).

d) Disturbed gas exchange of multifactorial etiology before/during/after birth. Extreme examples are: mechanical complications of delivery in a full-term fetus leading to stillbirth; immature lung parenchyma in a 24-week preterm newborn infant leading to neonatal death. On the other hand, a primary disturbance, such as toxicosis, may lead to death which, depending on the course, is given different diagnostic labels: dysmaturity, ablatio placenta, intrauterine asphyxia, postnatal asphyxia, immaturity, IRDS/hyaline membrane disease, or intra-cranial hemorrhage.

e) Postnatal infections (examples: sepsis, meningitis, bronchopneumonia, gastroenteritis).

Within each of the above groups, the most commonly used diagnoses are reported separately. There are several diagnoses, not only within the groups, but also between the groups, which overlap, or where differentiation is either difficult, not possible, or may depend on different criteria or different degrees of affect. In the data analyzed here, the following intermediate overlapping groups are used:

a) Intra-cranial hemorrhage: May be of hypoxic or traumatic origin.

b) Convulsions: May be intra-cranial hemorrhage/lesion, or sepsis/meningitis, or metabolic disorders.

c) Maceration of the fetus: may be embryopathy, fetopathy, or disturbed gas exchange, but signifies death at least some days before labor/delivery.

d) Unknown/no information: Total lack of helpful information is a real possibility in this kind of analysis and has to be accepted by having a group so labelled.

Table II. Functional causes of perinatal deaths

		Overlap	Symbols in figures	
Neonatal deaths	No information			
Embryofetopathy	Malformation		X	
	Fetopathy		•	
	Gastroenteritis		GE	
Infection	Broncopneumonia		Bp	
	Sepsis/meningitis		S	
Birth trauma	Convulsions		C	
	Intracranial — Lesion / bleeding			
	IRDS/HMD		H	
Disturbed respiratory adaptation	RDS		R	Disturbed gas exchange
	Apnea repetens		AR	
	Immaturity		I	
	Postpartum asphyxia			
Birth Stillbirths	Intrauterine asphyxia			
Complications of labor and delivery	Disproportion Presentation anomalies Cord anomalies Other complications		D	
	Ablatio placentae		A	
	Toxicosis/eclampsia		T	
	No maceration — no information			
	Maceration			
Complications of pregnancy	Placental infarction		P	
	Fetopathy		•	
	Embryopathy		X	

These groups have been arranged *in the most common sequence of time of death* around birth (table II). Disturbed gas exchange in stillbirths and neonatal deaths will form the center, with embryopathy and fetopathy repeated at the periphery of both stillbirths and neonatal deaths. The separate diagnoses within the main groups are also arranged in time sequence. At the same time, the aim has been to place the most commonly overlapping diagnoses as close to each other as possible. The most likely possibilities of overlapping are indicated in table II. Symbols that are used in the figures for the main groups are also given.

In this kind of analysis, *differentiation between stillbirth and early neonatal death* is, in some cases, difficult and must be borne in mind. Even with using the WHO criteria for live birth, there are situations in which 'alive' or 'dead' may be used interchangeably. A special situation may also arise for a pair of twins with a gestational age below 28 weeks, one having died before birth and thus an abortion, and the other having shown signs of life at birth but having died within 1 h, and thus a live birth with an early neonatal death. In such a perinatal study, only one of a twin pair may then be included in the analysis, as is the case in the present study.

Evaluation of growth, development, and maturity status at birth. As is well known and shown in all perinatal surveys, including this one, indices of maturity level of the fetus/newborn infant are heavily influencing the outcome. A functional analysis of causes of perinatal deaths, therefore, requires further dimensions for the evaluation of growth, development, and maturity of the fetus/newborn infant. These involve progress through the immediate perinatal period. Depending on the available information, such evaluation, however, has to be done at different levels.

Birth weight is the commonest recorded related variable and is used in groups of 250 g, with group medians of 750, 1,000, 1,250, 1,500 g, etc. (section III), as the basic, although crude, indicators of growth and development status at birth, and indirectly, to some extent, on the level of maturity.

Gestational age is a more direct indicator on the level of maturity, but gives primarily only a time concept. It has been recommended for use in crude grouping in *preterm* (less than 37 completed weeks), *full-term* (37–41 weeks), and *post-term* (equal or more than 42 weeks) (*Neligan et al.,* 1970). In this study, however, the gestational age, when known, will be grouped in each completed week hopefully improving the utilization of this variable.

The *relationship between variables* makes possible further estimations: birth weight and birth length in relation to gestational age as an indicator of intrauterine growth rate; birth weight and head circumference in relation to birth length as an indicator of the quality of intrauterine growth.

The evaluation of growth and development needs a reference frame. In the present study, a Swedish newborn growth chart constructed primarily from the Göteborg data has been used with birth weight and birth length against gestational age, and birth weight and head circumference against birth length. The basic principle has been to use the normally distributed main bulk of the population within each subgroup each week for gestational age, and each centimeter for birth length. We have used Göteborg data since they consist of a significantly larger number of completely measured newborn infants than in the Palermo material, and it has also been possible to secure values from Swedish national data, 1956–57 and 1973–74.

The differences between the two birth populations from Göteborg and Palermo (section III) are small in relation to the differences within each sample. Therefore, it is thought justified to use this Swedish newborn growth chart as a common base (section VI), though clearly the Palermo data are judged on the Swedish standards.

Procedure

The records of each case were scrutinized by two of us (P.K. and A.P.), and each case was given a single functional cause of death according to table II. No difficulties were experienced, realizing the possibility of overlapping diagnoses. For example, between IRDS and intracranial hemorrhage, and intracranial hemorrhage and convulsions. On the other hand, convulsions could also overlap with sepsis/meningitis, and so form an intermediate group.

Results

Functional causes of deaths. The incidences of *the perinatal diagnoses,* with sex differentiation, are given in table III. As in most perinatal surveys, there are more boys than girls. Since no clear difference of patterns was found (except for a slight tendency for girls to be more immature), the sexes were combined in the subsequent analysis. Since the two birth populations from which the deaths are obtained are of the same order of size, the absolute figures for deaths have primarily been used. There are $3^{1}/_{2}$ times as many deaths in Palermo as in Göteborg.

There are clear differences in the distribution pattern of applicable diagnoses between the two centers. In Palermo, there is a greater number of less-differentiated diagnoses, such as intrauterine asphyxia, asphyxia postpartum, and RDS (129, 37, and 87, respectively), than in Göteborg (1, 0, and 0, respectively). On the other hand, there is only one case of IRDS in Palermo compared to 23 in Göteborg. In Göteborg, IRDS with intraventricular hemorrhage is placed in the IRDS group. In Palermo, there are 29 intracranial hemorrhage cases that have been recognized as the main cause of death. However, how many of these were caused by hypoxia and how many by trauma is not possible to

Table III. Functional causes of deaths in relation to sex: stillbirths, early and late neonatal deaths

Diagnosis	Palermo										Göteborg			
	females		males		unknown sex		unknown place b. weight		total		EN		total	
	EN	LN	EN	LN	EN	LN	EN	LN	EN	LN	fe-males	males	EN	LN
Neonatal deaths														
No information	5	8	2	2	1				8	10				
Malformations														
Multiple malform. + trisomy 21	3	2	0	1					3	3	3	8	11	
CNS														
Heart/great vessels	1	1		4					1	5	1	4	5	2
Others and suspected	4	1	1	4					5	5	1	4	5	1
Fetopathies														
Prenatal infections											1	2	3	
Diabetes			2	4					2	4				
Hemolytic disease													0	1
Gastroenteritis		12	2	19	1		1	5	4	36				
Broncopneumonia	2	11	4	13			1	1	7	25		1	1	
Sepsis/meningitis	2	13	2	15			4	2	8	30	1	1	2	1
Convulsions		2	3	2			1	1	4	5				
Intracranial lesion			1				1		2		1	4	5	
Intracranial bleeding	6	6	10	6			1		17	12		5	5	1

IRDS/HMD	25				62	7	14	21
RDS					71			
Apnea repetens					1			
Immature					27			
Asphyxia postpartum					37			
Total early neonatal deaths	75	94	9	20	198	27	51	78
Total late neonatal deaths	66	76		9	151			8
Total neonatal deaths	141	170	9	29	349	27	51	86

Birth

Stillbirths								
Intrauterine asphyxia	53	68	7	1	129	4	8	12
Complicated delivery	1				1		1	1
Ablatio placentae	1	1			2	5	8	13
Toxicosis/eclampsia						2	6	8
No maceration	47	51	18	4	120	2	2	4
Maceration	6	4			10	13	9	22
Placental infarction					0	6	2	8
Fetopathies	3	4			7	4	2	6
Embryopathies	6	2			8	3	2	5
Total stillbirths	117	130	25	5	277	39	40	79
Total stillbirths and neonatal deaths	258	300	34	34	626	66	91	165

EN = Early; LN = late neonatal deaths; ST = stillbirths.

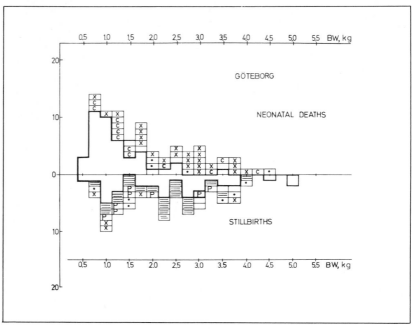

Fig. 2. Göteborg. The individual cases of stillbirths and neonatal deaths in relation to birth weight groups of 250 g. Symbols as in table II.

determine from the available information. There are about the same number of malformations in Palermo and Göteborg – 26 and 29, respectively. In the case of postnatal infections, on the other hand, there are 110 in Palermo and 4 in Göteborg.

Main functional causes of deaths in relation to birth weight groups of 250 g. In figures 2 and 3, the individual cases in the main groups have been related graphically to the birth weight groups of 250 g. In Göteborg, the gas-exchange disturbances below birth weight 1,375 g dominate with a tail towards the higher birth weights as stillbirths. The neonatal deaths within the higher birth weights are mostly malformations or fetopathies. These diagnoses seem to be dominant in stillbirths for the small fetuses. Palermo shows a similar pattern for the very small fetuses to that in Göteborg, but there is a higher prevalence of gas-exchange disturbances as the cause of neonatal death in all birth weight groups, and a large number of them among the stillbirths around 3.5 kg birth weight. There is a clear two-population distribution. There are postnatal infections scattered over all birth weights. Malformations and fetopathies show about the same pattern as in Göteborg.

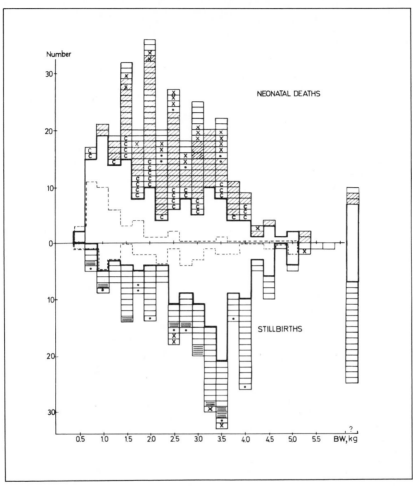

Fig. 3. Palermo. The individual cases of stillbirths and neonatal deaths in relation to birth weight groups of 250 g. Symbols as in table II. Gas-exchange disturbances of Göteborg are enclosed by the broken line.

The early and late neonatal deaths are combined in the analysis of the *different places of confinement* in the two centers. The distribution of applicable diagnoses is given in table IV. In figures 4—11, the relationships to birth weight are shown graphically, and the separate diagnoses are also indicated.

In figures 2—11, cases with gas-exchange disturbances are enclosed by the heavy line (table II).

Table IV. Functional causes of deaths in relation to place of delivery: stillbirths and neonatal deaths

Diagnosis	Place of delivery							
	Palermo						Göteborg	
	Univ. Hosp.	Hosp. A	Hosp. B	Hosp. A or B	Priv. clin.	home deliv.	West Hosp.	East Hosp.
Neonatal deaths								
No information	2	7	6		2	1		
Malformations								
Multiple malform. + trisomy 21	3		1		1	1	6	5
CNS								
Heart/great vessels	1				1		2	5
Others and suspect	2	3	2		3		3	3
Fetopathies								
Prenatal infections							1	2
Diabetes			4			1	1	
Hemolytic disease								
Gastroenteritis	1	14	6	2	7	4		
Broncopneumonia	4	8	5		6	7	1	
Sepsis/meningitis	3	10	6		10	3		2
Convulsions	1	5		1				
Intracranial lesion	1	1					2	4
Intracranial bleeding	1	8	5		7	7	1	5

IRDS/HMD	11	1		6	14	14	13	9
RDS		23	13				1	2
Apnea repetens	2				5	1		
Immature	3	13					8	9
Asphyxia postpartum	3	12	7		12	6		
Total early neonatal deaths								
Total late neonatal deaths								
Total neonatal deaths	37	105	55	9	69	45	39	47
Birth								
Stillbirths								
Intrauterine asphyxia	14	42	18	14	21	19	5	1
Complicated delivery	1						7	7
Ablatio placentae	1					1	6	6
Toxicosis/eclampsia								2
No maceration	15	36	26	10	17	12	3	1
Maceration		5		3		2	13	9
Placenta infarction			1	1	2		4	4
Fetopathies	2	3	1	1			6	1
Empryopathies	3					1	4	
Total stillbirths	36	86	46	29	40	35	48	31
Total stillbirths and neonatal deaths	73	191	101	38	109	80	87	78
Total births with known birth weights	1,032	1,510	1,293	630	4,908	3,156	5,585	6,686

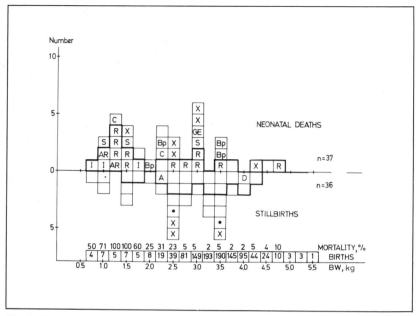

Fig. 4. Palermo University Hospital. The individual cases of stillbirths and neonatal deaths in relation to birth weight groups of 250 g for the different places of birth. Symbols as in table II.

Fig. 5. Palermo Hospital A. The individual cases of stillbirths and neonatal deaths in relation to birth weight groups of 250 g for the different places of births. Symbols as in table II.

Fig. 6. Palermo Hospital B. The individual cases of stillbirths and neonatal deaths in relation to birth weight groups of 250 g for the different places of births. Symbols as in table II.

Fig. 7. Palermo Hospital A *or* B. The individual cases of stillbirths and neonatal deaths in relation to birth weight groups of 250 g for the different places of births. Symbols as in table II.

Fig. 8. Palermo private clinics. The individual cases of stillbirths and neonatal deaths in relation to birth weight groups of 250 g for the different places of births. Symbols as in table II.

Fig. 9. Palermo home delivery. The individual cases of stillbirths and neonatal deaths in relation to birth weight groups of 250 g for the different places of births. Symbols as in table II.

Fig. 10. Göteborg West Hospital. The individual cases of stillbirths and neonatal deaths in relation to birth weight groups of 250 g for the different places of births. Symbols as in table II.

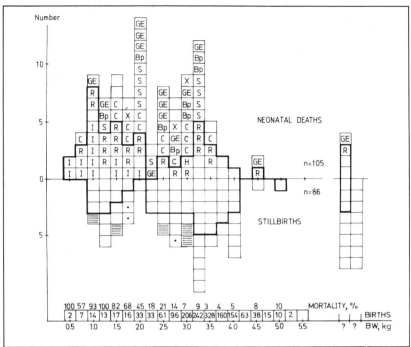

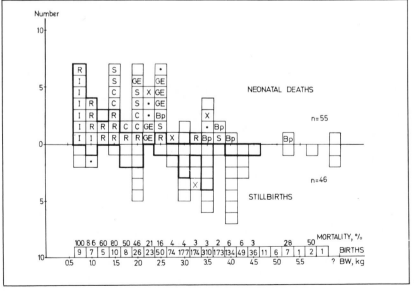

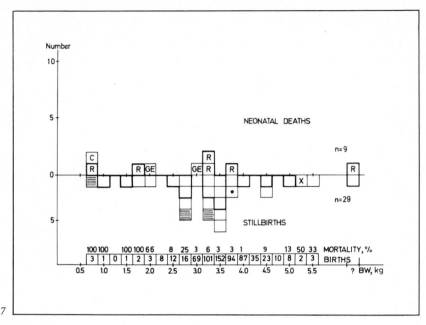

7

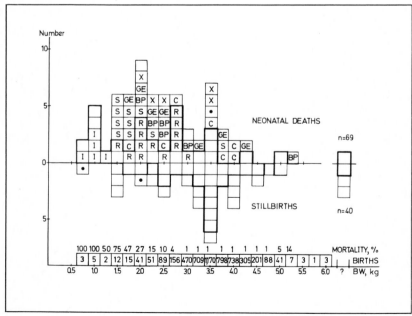

8

For legends, see p. 100.

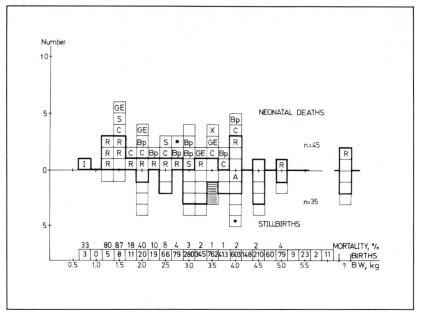

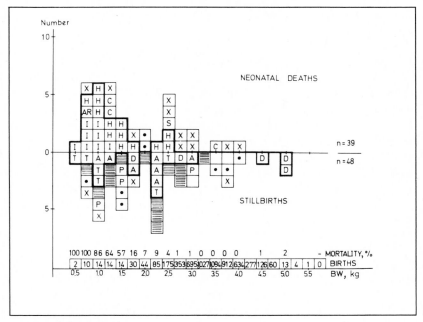

For legends, see p. 100.

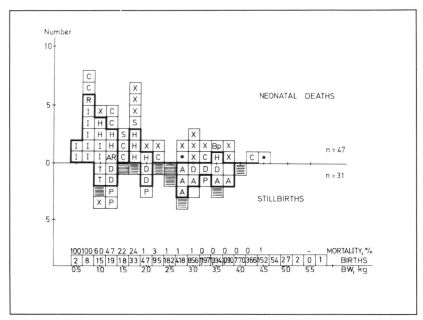

Fig. 11. Göteborg East Hospital. The individual cases of stillbirths and neonatal deaths in relation to birth weight groups of 250 g for the different places of births. Symbols as in table II.

Evaluation of growth and development, and maturity status, at birth. In figures 12–15, graphical presentations are given of the relationships of birth-weight and birth length to gestational age, and of the relationships of birth weight and head circumference to birth length for stillbirths and neonatal deaths (early and late) in the Göteborg and the Palermo materials. As a background reference the distributions of the Göteborg material are used. In the birth weight/gestational age relationship the two sexes are separated, boys: unbroken lines; girls: broken lines. The justification of the clinical use of the Göteborg reference also for the Palermo material is discussed above and in section VI.

The birth weight/gestational age relationship, clinically mostly used. In Göteborg, the stillbirths are dominated by light-for-date fetuses, i.e. retarded intrauterine growth (38% below − 2 SD; 61% below − 1 SD, expected 2.5 and 17%, respectively), and mostly showing embryopathy, fetopathy or maceration. Stillbirths among fetuses whose weights were appropriate for gestational age are mostly related to acute delivery complications. When born alive after 34 weeks of gestation and without malformation, practically all newborn babies survive the neonatal period. Among those born before 34 weeks of gestation, the hazard increases with low gestational age and more than one third of these neonatal deaths were below 28 weeks of gestation. The weight of most of the newborn infants below 34 weeks was appropriate for gestational age.

In Palermo, the stillbirths are found mostly among appropriate- and heavy-for-gestational-age fetuses above 34 weeks of gestation chiefly due to intrauterine asphyxia. As in Göteborg, the neonatal deaths are found firstly among the appropriate-for-gestational-age newborn infants below 33 weeks of gestation, but then spread out. Malformations occur primarily as in Göteborg among the full-term infants. Among the gas exchange disturbances or infections, there are several both light-for-date and heavy-for-date babies.

The birth weight/birth length relationships. In the Göteborg material, there is an intriguing shift towards light-for-length, most pronounced among the stillbirths. In perinatal deaths, with a birth weight above 1,250 g and with measured birth length of the stillbirths, only six were above, but 44 below the birth weight for given birth length; and of the neonatal deaths, only five were above but 50 below. In Palermo, the birth length was available only in a restricted number of stillbirths (16%). However, some of the fetuses who died by gas-exchange disturbances were extremely heavy for given birth length. The same holds for the neonatal deaths (31% measured); but also for infants with a birth weight of 1,000–2,000 g, there is the same tendency. On the other hand, there is a dominance among infants with postnatal infections with a birth weight above 2,000 g to be light-for-given-birth length. The smallest preterm infants seem to have an appropriate relationship.

The birth length/gestational age relationship. In Göteborg, there is no clear differentiation as was expected since birth weight shows a tendency to be low for both gestational age and for birth length. In Palermo, the full-term neonatal deaths are, as a group, shorter for age in spite of a very similar cumulative distribution of birth length in the total birth population, which is in conformity with a tendency towards overweight in relation to length.

The head circumference/birth length relationship. Head circumference is virtually only available in the Göteborg data. The relationship shows in general a proportional growth against length, however, also here limited numbers (56%).

The *cause of infant deaths between 4 weeks and 1 year* are given in table V. In Palermo, infections dominate, while in Göteborg, malformations and sudden death are most frequent. The percentage incidence of the main groups of diagnoses in relation to time of death is given in table VI.

Discussion

This method of evaluation of the functional causes of perinatal deaths, including late neonatal deaths, has been designed to be applicable to different perinatal information systems with varying 'hardness' and 'softness' of primary

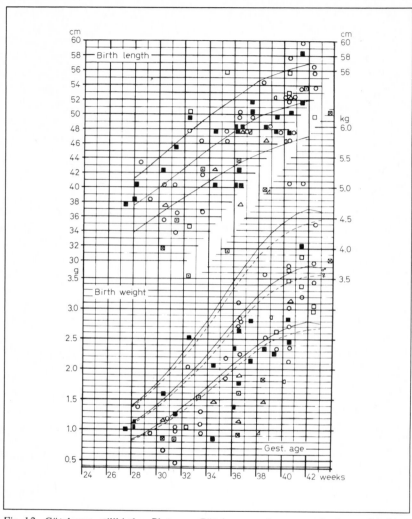

12a

Fig. 12. Göteborg: stillbirths. Plots on Göteborg newborn growth chart with birth weight and birth length against gestational age and birth weight and head circumference against birth length.

data (section II). The main purposes of such a system are to reveal the main hazards within systems of perinatal care, to indicate the need for more detailed studies, and/or to concentrate resources in specific areas. In clinical practice, one can also, within a short period of time, see potential changing patterns of emerging problems and then adjust curative regimens.

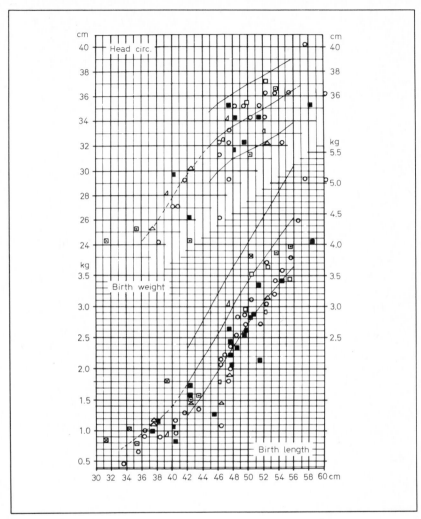

12b

Although the method has been developed upon the data base of the joint study, there is reason to believe that it is applicable to a variety of study designs. In the present study, methods used for collecting primary data represent two extremes: a prospective method, forming part of the clinical work in a standardized system of perinatal care; and an early retrospective method (24 h to 7 days)

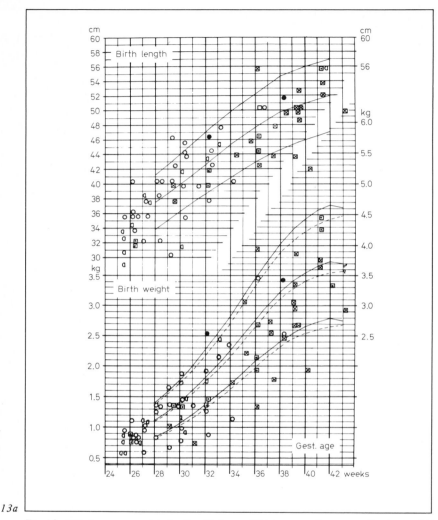

13a

Fig. 13. Göteborg: neonatal deaths. Plots on Göteborg newborn growth chart with birth weight and birth length against gestational age and birth weight and head circumference against birth length.

applied to greatly differing systems of perinatal care, carried out by a small team working in a society with limited experience of this kind of research. For the main conclusions, related and overlapping diagnoses are grouped together, and intermediate overlapping groups have been formed. As long as these latter groups are relatively small, or show the same pattern, their presence is acceptable.

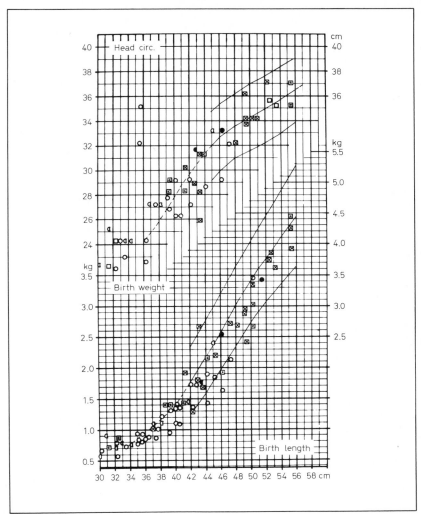

13b

Furthermore, uncertainty in differentiation, in some cases, between stillbirth and early neonatal death will be reduced in influence. The second dimension, birth weight in 250-gram groups, gives an essential differentiation.

The application of this method of evaluation of the FCD to the data of the first Report of the British Perinatal Survey (*Butler and Bonham,* 1963) is shown

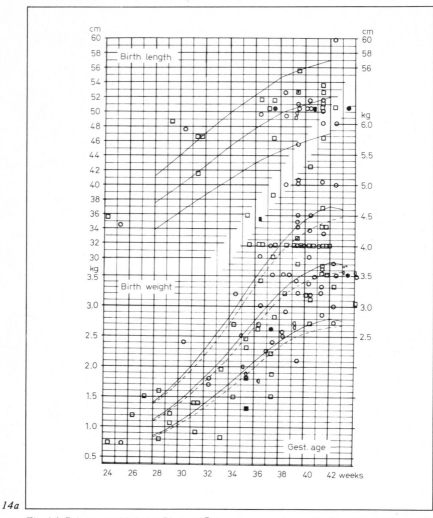

14a

Fig. 14. Palermo: stillbirths. Plots on Palermo newborn growth chart with birth weight and birth length against gestational age and birth weight and head circumference against birth length.

in figure 16, where the birth weight is grouped as reported in the above survey in the following three main groups: < 1 kg; between 1 and 2.5 kg, and > 2.5 kg.

The analysis indicates clearly that the main perinatal hazards in Göteborg are small newborn infants failing to make the necessary gas exchange adaptation;

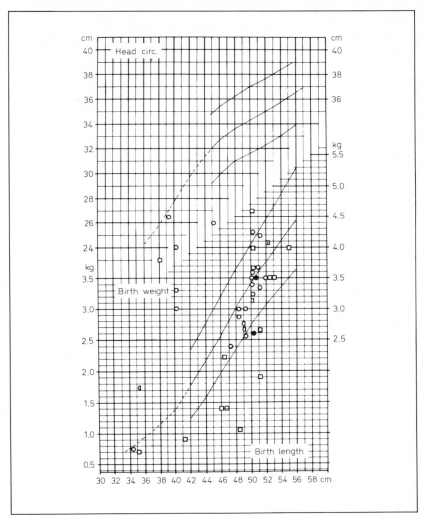

14b

full-term newborn infants with functionally significant malformations and feto-pathies, and stillbirths due to toxicosis, ablatio placenta and other complications of delivery (6 per 1,000). The same perinatal hazards are present in Palermo, but there is also a high risk of disturbed gas exchange among the full-term newborn infants, and the risk of stillbirths is 3–4 times higher. The findings indicate a

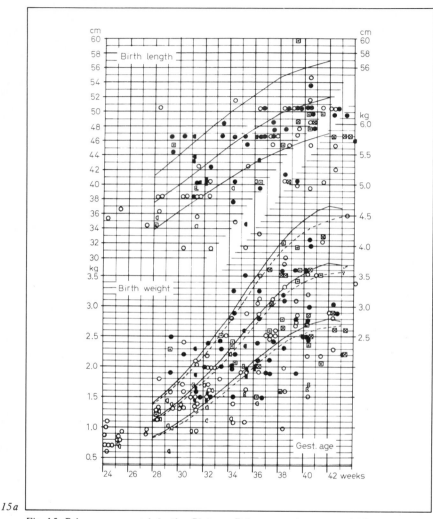

15a

Fig. 15. Palermo: neonatal deaths. Plots on Palermo newborn growth chart with birth weight and birth length against gestational age and birth weight and head circumference against birth length.

two-population distribution, one for the small fetuses/newborn infants, and one for the larger ones with a dividing line around 2,250 g. Postnatal infections play an important superimposed role for neonatal mortality here.

In Göteborg, there is no clear difference in pattern between the two hospitals, though there is a tendency towards a higher incidence of low birth weight

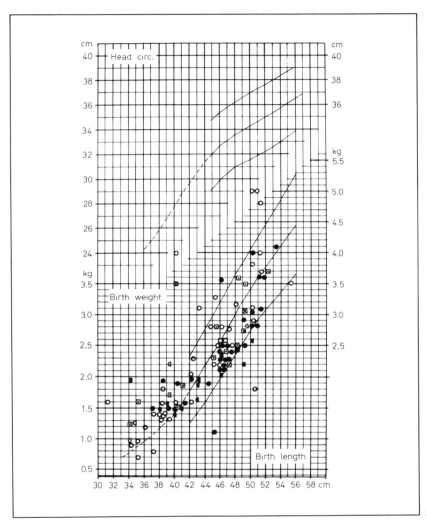

15b

stillbirths in the West hospital. The limited number of cases does not allow any general conclusions.

In Palermo, however, there are big differences between the different places of confinement as illustrated in the figures. Hospital A shows the most pronounced two-population trend.

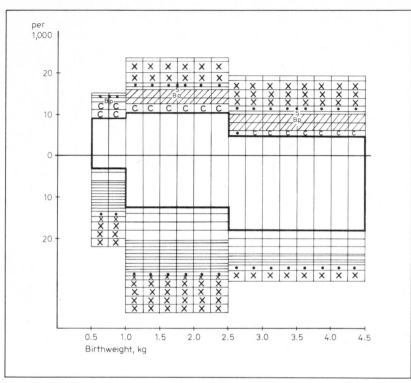

Fig. 16. The described method of grouping by main functional causes of death and birth weight, in relation to birth weight groups as applied to the British Perinatal Survey (*Butler and Bonham,* 1963).

When evaluation of intrauterine growth was included, further information was obtained. The relationship between birth weight and gestational age is schematically indicated in figure 17. In Göteborg, the stillbirths are in general characterized by being light-for-dates, irrespective of the main cause. The neonatal deaths, with a gestational age of 34 weeks or more, are practically all malformations, some are light-for-date, and some are not. Most of the neonatal deaths below 34 weeks are appropriate-for-dates, a few light-for-dates. Follow-up studies reported elsewhere indicate that survivors with later sequelae are found mostly among the light-for-dates babies (*Sabel et al.,* 1976; *Kjellmer et al.,* 1976).

In Palermo, most of the stillbirths are full-term infants with several heavy-for-dates. The light-for-date babies are found among the neonatal deaths, mostly with a gestational age of 34 weeks or more. There are also quite a few heavy-for-dates. The majority, however, are in the middle stream which is the dominant

Table V. Functional causes of deaths in relation to place of delivery: infant deaths 28 days to 11 months

Diagnosis	Place of delivery									
	Palermo							Göteborg		
	Univ. Hosp.	Hosp. A	Hosp. B	Priv. clin.	home deliv.	un-known	total	West Hosp.	East Hosp.	total
Malformations										
Multiple malform. + trisomy 21	1			3	1		5	1	1	2
CNS										
Heart/great vessels								1	3	4
Others									4	4
Hereditary disease									1	1
Hematological disease									1	1
Digestive system disease						1	1			
Infections										
Gastroenteritis		3		1	6		10	1	1	2
Bronchopneumonia		6	5	5	6	1	23	2	1	3
Sepsis/meningitis		1		2			3			
Others					1		1			
Heart failure		1			3		4			
Respiratory disorders										
Apnoea repetens									1	1
Pneumothorax									1	1
Sudden deaths									6	6
No information				1			1			
Total	1	11	5	12	17	2	48	5	20	25

Table VI. Functional causes of death in relation to age of death

Diagnosis	Age of death																	
	0–11 hrs		12–23 hrs		24–27 hrs		2–6 days		7–13 days		14–20 days		21–27 days		28d–1 yr		0–1 yr	
	n	%	n	%	n	%	n	%	n	%	n	%	n	%	n	%	n	%
Göteborg																		
No information																		
Malformations	6	25	2	33	4	24	9	29	3	50					10	40	34	31
Fetopathies	2	8							1	17							4	4
Postnatal infect.			1	17			2	6			1	100			5	20	9	8
Convulsions																		
Intracran. lesion					2	12	8	26	2	33							12	11
Intracran. bleed.																		
IRDS/HMD	3	13	2	33	10	59	9	29					1	100			25	23
RDS																		
Apnea repetens																		
Immaturitas	13	54	1	17	1	6	2	6									17	15
Asphyxia postpart.																		
Respir. disorders															8	32	8	7
Heart failure																		
Digest. syst. disease															2	8	2	2
Total	24	100	6	100	17	100	31	100	6	100	1	100	1	100	25	100	111	100

Palermo

	1 n	1 %	2 n	2 %	3 n	3 %	4 n	4 %	5 n	5 %	6 n	6 %	7 n	7 %	8 n	8 %	Total n	Total %
No information	3	5	2	7	2	4	1	2	7	11	3	6	1	3	1	2	19	5
Malformations	4	7	1	4	1	2	3	5	4	6	4	7	1	3	5	10	23	6
Fetopathies							1	2	1	2	3	6					6	2
Postnatal infect.			1	4	1	2	17	27	30	48	36	67	25	71	37	77	147	37
Convulsions	4	7	3	10	8	17	8	13	6	10			6	17			40	10
Intracran. lesion																		
Intracran. bleed.																		
IRDS/HMD RDS	12	20	14	50	23	49	24	38	12	19	5	9					90	23
Apnea repetens																		
Immaturitas	9	15	3	10	6	13	9	14	2	3	3	6	2	6			30	8
Asphyxia postpart.	27	46	4	14	5	11	1	2			3	6	1	3			37	9
Respir. disorders																		
Heart failure															4	8	4	1
Digest. syst. disease															1	2	1	0.3
Total	59	100	28	100	47	100	64	100	62	100	54	100	35	100	48	100	397	100

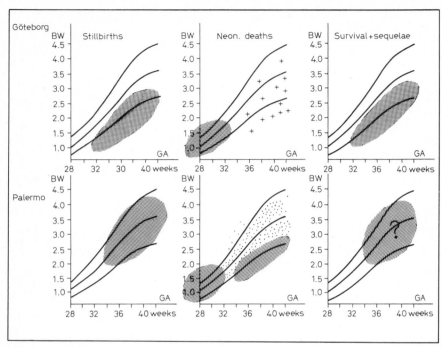

Fig. 17. Risk areas in the relationship birth weight/gestational age for stillbirths and neonatal deaths in Göteborg and Palermo, and for survivors with sequelae in Göteborg.

feature of the smallest infants. There is no information in Palermo available with respect to survivors with sequelae.

The relationship of birth weight to gestational age reflects intrauterine growth rate. The relationship of birth weight to birth length introduces a new dimension, and it reflects the quality of intrauterine growth. Hyponutrition or hypernutrition may also be differentiated.

In Göteborg, all perinatal deaths with birth weights from 1,250 g, regardless of cause of death, have a low birth weight in relation to mean weight for given birth length, indicating intrauterine hyponutrition. In Palermo, intrauterine hyponutrition seems to indicate susceptibility to postnatal infection. On the other hand, intrauterine hypernutrition seems to have a significant impact for gas-exchange disturbance around birth for the full-term infants, possibly as a mechanical factor. Whether hypernutrition and accelerated intrauterine growth have an influence on the etiology of very preterm infants of 24–26 weeks gestation is an open question. The relationship of birth weight to birth length seems to be of great importance in the perinatal field reflecting situations of negative effect at both poles of the distribution. It has the advantage of calculation from two direct body measurements. Gestational age is not involved — a variable which can always introduce a potential error.

Conclusions

In *both cities,* there are the problems, of the same magnitude, of preterm deliveries of small, immature babies. In Göteborg, the perinatal mortality is dominated by retarded intrauterine growth and intrauterine hyponutrition caused by embryopathy or fetopathies of different kinds. The importance of this is further stressed by the relationship to survivors with sequelae (reported elsewhere). The comparatively total small number of deaths in Göteborg must be noted.

In Palermo, postnatal infections are of significant importance. Here, retarded intrauterine growth, and especially intrauterine hyponutrition, seem to be related to susceptibility to such infections. On the other hand, accelerated intrauterine growth and hypernutrition seem to be a significantly contributory factor to a main problem in Palermo — gas-exchange disturbances in full-term infants, causing stillbirths or neonatal deaths, possibly as a mechanical mechanism.

Intrauterine growth rate and intrauterine nutrition are two factors certainly often related, but may not always be so. They both operate over a full range to extremes in positive and negative directions. As usual in biological events, there are probably no definite borderlines between health and pathological conditions, being an interplay with other factors in the multifactorial perinatal field. A continuous scale is the most useful tool allowing for wide variations. Characterization of the individual situation by deviation from corresponding mean values, expressed in fractions of standard deviations, is a useful method when Gaussian distribution is present; or, if not, after transformation (section VI). Finally, it has to be remarked that the relationship of cause of death to birth weight is subject to sampling errors. Of Palermo deaths, 12% have unknown birth weight.

Summary

A method of evaluating the functional cause of perinatal deaths is presented. The design is based on the use of perinatal information collected in different situations. Evaluation of intrauterine growth increases the efficacy of the method. Especially useful is the relationship between birth weight and birth length. When applied to deaths in the study in Palermo and Göteborg (respectively, 626 and 165), differing patterns were found between the two cities, and between the different places of deliveries in Palermo.

In Göteborg, factors leading to perinatal deaths seem, in a dominant fashion, to be associated with slow intrauterine growth and intrauterine under-nutrition. In Palermo, disturbed gas exchange during labor, delivery, and the immediate neonatal period, and

Karlberg/Priolisi/Landström/Selstam

postnatal infections, dominate the picture. The analyses indicate that intrauterine hypernutrition may play a role in the mechanism of the former situations, and intrauterine hyponutrition in the mechanism of the latter situations. Preterm deliveries with very small and immature babies are common to both Göteborg and Palermo. These findings form a basis for defining priority areas within perinatal care and for further research within the perinatal field.

Reference

Butler, N. and Bonham, D.: Perinatal mortality. The first report of the 1958 British perinatal mortality survey under the auspices of the National Birthday Trust Fund (Livingstone, Edinburgh 1963).

Kjellmer, I.; Andersson, U.B.; Aronson, M.; Karlberg, P.; Landström, T.; Liedholm, M., and Selstam, U.: Relation between risk factors in the neonatal period and later neurological and developmental disturbances. Abstract. 5th Eur. Congr. Perinatal Medicine, Uppsala, 1976.

Neligan, G.A., et al.: Working party to discuss nomenclature based on gestational age and birth weight. Proc. 2nd Eur. Congr. Perinatal Medicine, London 1970, pp. 172–173 (Karger, Basel 1971).

Sabel, K.G.; Olegård, R., and Victorin, L.: Remaining sequelae with modern perinatal care. Pediatrics, Springfield *57:* 652 (1976).

Smith, C.A. and Nelson, N.M.: The physiology of the newborn infant; 4th ed. (Ch.C. Thomas, Springfield 1976).

Prof. *P. Karlberg,* Department of Pediatrics, University of Göteborg, East Hospital, *S–416 85 Göteborg* (Sweden)
Prof. *A. Priolisi,* Child Health Institute, Palermo University, Via Lancia Dibrolo 10 B, *Palermo* (Italy)

Section V

Monogr. Paediat., vol. 9, pp. 121–164 (Karger, Basel 1977)

Measures of Maturity Indices in Perinatal Mortality

J.R. Ashford, J.G. Fryer, P. Karlberg, A. Priolisi and R.A. Harding

Department of Mathematical Statistics and Operational Research, University of Exeter, Exeter, Devon

I. Introduction

The analyses described in section I have shown that there are substantial differences in mortality rates between the two cities, as expected, and also between the various places of confinement. Mortality rates are closely related to birth weight, and it was found that within each city part, but not all, of these differences can be attributed to variations in the distribution of birth weight. In fact, *Fryer* (1976) has devised a simple method of measuring the importance of differing birth weight distributions, and here, the measure indicates that the difference in birth weight distributions accounts for a relatively small percentage of the difference in mortality rates. When the cause of death was considered, the excess of late neonatal mortality at Palermo appeared to be associated with infectious diseases, which had no significant impact upon mortality at Göteborg. These factors cover only a small part of the spectrum of biological, socio-economic, clinical and other characteristics which are known to influence perinatal and infant mortality. The purpose of the present paper is to examine the available evidence in greater depth, to ascertain the other factors involved and the extent to which they are associated with variations in mortality rates.

II. Perinatal Mortality and Indices of Maturity

The distribution of the various measures of maturity has been considered in detail in section III. In view of the evidence given in that paper concerning digit preference at 'round' numbers, the grouping of the data concerning maturity has been deliberately chosen to minimise this effect. The relation between perinatal mortality and birth weight in the two surveys for single births is presented in these terms in figure 1. For the reasons given in section I, a non-linear 'probit'

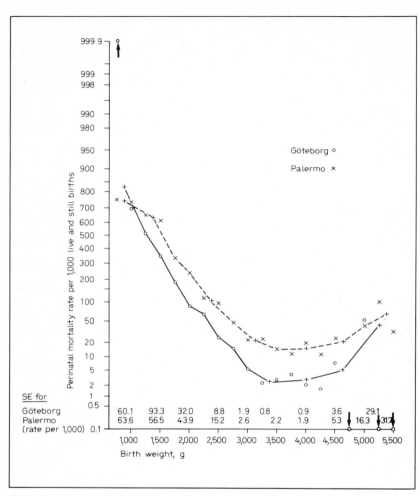

Fig. 1. Perinatal mortality in terms of birth weight (all single births).

scale has been chosen for the mortality measurement. Raw mortality rates are plotted using symbols like ⊙, ✕ and +. Some of the data points correspond to zero and 100% mortality. These are recorded at the limits of the graph and indicated by an arrow (↓ or ↑). In addition, we have tried to draw a single line indicating the general trend of the data and some adjacent groups have been combined to make it smoother.

To give an indication of the accuracy of the data points, estimates have been calculated of their respective standard errors, based upon the theory of binomial distribution which is approximately appropriate if not totally. The results obtained are indicated in the figure and are located immediately beneath the data points to which they refer. Just under half of the deaths taking place within the first 12 h of life in fact occur within the first hour. The standard error of the estimates of the mortality rate tends to decrease with increasing numbers of subjects and rate, and is therefore least for the most commonly occurring birth weights, between about 3,000 and 5,000 g.

Both relationships show the same general form, with a linear (on the probit scale) decrease in perinatal mortality with increasing birth weight up to about 3,000 g, a relatively constant rate between 3,000 and 4,000 g and a subsequent increase with increasing birth weight beyond 4,000 g. Apart from the very low birth weights, perinatal mortality at Palermo is substantially (and significantly) higher than at Göteborg throughout the range. The relative difference is greatest for birth weights of about 3,500 g (the median of the distribution), where the perinatal mortality rates are lowest − 2.5 per 1,000 live and still births at Göteborg and 14 per 1,000 at Palermo. Whilst birth weight was recorded for all the Göteborg births, this item was not available for some 622 (just under 5%) of the single births at Palermo. The perinatal mortality rate for this group was about 84 per 1,000, in comparison with 33 per 1,000 for the whole population. On this basis, it appears that the unknown birth weights cannot be regarded as a random sample and probably occur preferentially at the low end of the birth weight scale. However, in view of the comparatively small proportion of the population involved, it is considered that the available data provided a reasonably accurate representation of the underlying relationship between birth weight and perinatal mortality, apart from in the lowest birth weight groups.

The relation between perinatal mortality and gestational age is illustrated in figure 2, which has been plotted in the same way as figure 1. Information about gestational age is not available for all types of record at Palermo and the corresponding data refer to the edited standard records. The general trend of the results is similar on both surveys and closely resembles that for birth weight. For pregnancies of up to about 39 weeks, perinatal mortality falls linearly with gestational age (on the probit scale). As gestational age increases further, at Palermo mortality then shows a slight increase, but at Göteborg the rates remain effectively constant. In comparison with figure 1, the range of variation of perinatal mortality over the linear part of the mortality-maturity relation is somewhat smaller, as is the difference between the two surveys in this region. The largest relative differences between the surveys occur at and above the average gestational age (about 40 weeks). At Göteborg, the proportion of records with unknown gestational age was negligible, but at Palermo this item was not available for some 168 (3.6%) of the edited standard records. Perinatal mortality in this group was 77 per 1,000, compared with 33 per 1,000 for the complete population. On this basis, it is likely that the records with unknown gestational

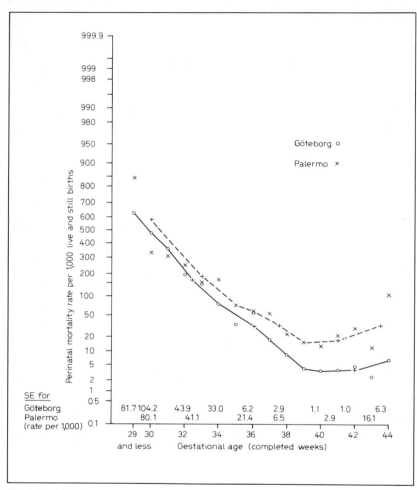

Fig. 2. Perinatal mortality in terms of gestational age (all single births).

age were drawn selectively from the lower part of the range of maturity. However, in view of the small proportion of records involved, the relation between perinatal mortality and gestational age is not likely to have been seriously affected, though perhaps bias is a factor in the lowest gestational age groups.

The results for the third measure of maturity, birth length, are presented in figure 3, the data for Palermo again being based upon the edited standard records. The general trends are similar to those for birth weight and gestation. However, the tendency for mortality to increase at the upper end of the scale is

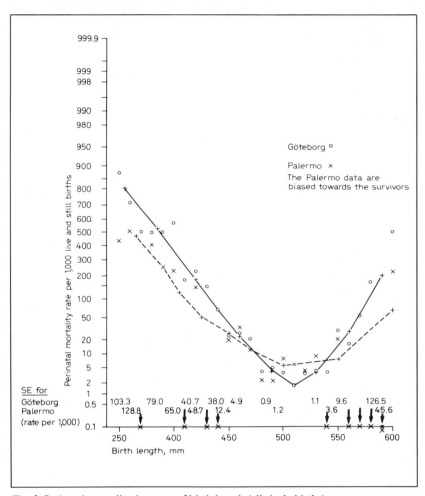

Fig. 3. Perinatal mortality in terms of birth length (all single births).

considerably more marked. In contrast to figures 1 and 2, Palermo appears to be
at a clear advantage over Göteborg at both the lower and the upper parts of the
scale. On the other hand, mortality in the range between 490 and 540 mm
(which covers the majority of both populations) is lower at Göteborg, although
the differences in mortality in the central part of the distribution are considerably smaller than those for birth weight or gestation. However, the fact that
Palermo appears in a better light in this analysis can be attributed to the effect
of excluding observations with unknown birth length. Although only some 300

(6.4%) of the edited standard records are involved, perinatal mortality in this group was as high as 357 per 1,000. Thus, by excluding records with unknown birth length, substantial numbers of the perinatal deaths were also omitted and there is little doubt that the trends shown in figure 3 underestimate the levels of perinatal mortality at Palermo at both the lower and the upper parts of the scale. At Göteborg, birth length was recorded for all except 26 (0.2%) of the single births and, although there were 10 perinatal deaths (385 per 1,000) in this group, the bias is much less marked.

A fourth measure of maturity, head circumference, is available only for Göteborg, and the relation with perinatal mortality was examined. The general trend of the results is similar to that of figures 1–3, with mortality falling linearly as head circumference increases, reaching a minimum and subsequently showing a slight increase at the upper end of the scale. Although head circumference was recorded for all except 157 single births (1.4%) at Göteborg, the group included 70 out of the 134 perinatal deaths. For this reason, the analysis should be regarded as merely providing a general indication of the probable trends in the whole population and the results have not been included in this paper.

In summary, when each of the measures of maturity is taken singly, perinatal mortality amongst single births shows a wide variation with 'maturity' (birth weight): from 600–800 per 1,000 for the most immature to 2–3 per 1,000 at Göteborg and 6–20 per 1,000 at Palermo in the region of the centre of the distribution of maturity. The general similar of the forms of the relationships for the different measures of maturity is consistent with birth weight, gestational age, birth length and head circumference being moderately well correlated. Each individual measure reflects what might be termed the 'general maturity' of the infant and the latter is in turn closely associated with perinatal mortality. However, the correlation is by no means perfect and the relation between mortality, and two or more measures considered jointly is also of interest. The numbers of multiple births on either survey are insufficient to permit a similar set of analyses for this group.

III. Perinatal Mortality and Multiple Measures of Maturity

Of the four measures of maturity, we have seen that the relationships between birth length and perinatal mortality at Palermo and between head circumference and perinatal mortality at Göteborg are biassed because of the selective omission of data. For this reason, analysis of the joint measures of maturity has been confined mainly to birth weight and gestation, the data for Palermo being based upon the edited standard records. In the first place we have considered the relationship between perinatal mortality and one of these two measures for given

Table I. Perinatal mortality in terms of birth weight and gestational age, all single births. Rate per 1,000 live and still-births

Birth weight g	Gestational age, completed weeks											unknown	Total
	≤ 32	33	34	35	36	37	38	39	40	41	42 or more		
(a) Göteborg													
≤ 875	1,000 (15)	– (0)	1,000 (1)	– (0)	– (0)	– (0)	– (0)	– (0)	– (0)	– (0)	– (0)	1,000 (1)	1,000 (17)
876– 1,375	606 (33)	500 (6)	500 (2)	– (0)	750 (4)	– (0)	– (0)	0 (1)	– (0)	– (0)	– (0)	750 (4)	600 (50)
1,376– 1,875	258 (31)	250 (8)	125 (8)	143 (7)	400 (5)	250 (4)	333 (6)	0 (2)	– (0)	– (0)	– (0)	250 (4)	240 (75)
1,876– 2,375	125 (16)	77 (13)	50 (20)	83 (24)	130 (23)	51 (39)	77 (13)	63 (32)	130 (23)	0 (8)	0 (7)	0 (14)	73 (232)
2,376– 2,875	143 (14)	0 (9)	0 (20)	0 (53)	52 (77)	30 (101)	18 (169)	15 (201)	18 (166)	0 (114)	0 (80)	19 (53)	19 (1,057)
2,876– 3,375	0 (3)	0 (4)	125 (8)	0 (20)	0 (75)	5 (200)	0 (388)	4 (830)	1 (947)	3 (626)	9 (460)	7 (148)	4 (3,709)
3,376– 3,875	500 (2)	0 (1)	0 (5)	0 (9)	0 (34)	12 (85)	7 (291)	1 (835)	2 (1,244)	3 (956)	4 (783)	6 (168)	3 (4,413)
3,876– 4,375	– (0)	– (0)	0 (1)	333 (3)	200 (5)	0 (23)	0 (80)	0 (261)	0 (587)	4 (559)	0 (474)	0 (54)	2 (2,047)

Continued on next page.

Table I (continued)

Birth weight g	Gestational age, completed weeks												Total
	≤32	33	34	35	36	37	38	39	40	41	42 or more	unknown	
4,376–4,875	– (0)	– (0)	– (0)	0 (2)	– (0)	0 (3)	0 (11)	0 (37)	0 (95)	9 (114)	9 (109)	0 (20)	5 (391)
4,876–5,375	– (0)	– (0)	– (0)	– (0)	– (0)	– (0)	0 (2)	0 (3)	143 (7)	71 (14)	0 (19)	0 (1)	43 (46)
5,376 or more	– (0)	– (0)	– (0)	– (0)	– (0)	– (0)	0 (1)	– (0)	– (0)	– (0)	0 (1)	– (0)	0 (2)
Unknown	– (0)	– (0)	– (0)	– (0)	– (0)	– (0)	– (0)	– (0)	– (0)	– (0)	– (0)	– (0)	– (0)
Total	421 (114)	146 (41)	77 (65)	34 (118)	58 (223)	18 (455)	8 (961)	4 (2,202)	4 (3,069)	4 (2,391)	4 (1,933)	17 (467)	11 (12,039)

(b) Palermo (edited standard records)

≤875	833 (6)	1,000 (1)	– (0)	– (0)	– (0)	– (0)	– (0)	– (0)	– (0)	– (0)	– (0)	1,000 (1)	875 (8)
876–1,375	818 (11)	– (0)	– (0)	1,000 (1)	– (0)	0 (1)	– (0)	– (0)	– (0)	– (0)	– (0)	1,000 (3)	812 (16)
1,376–1,875	500 (16)	250 (4)	500 (4)	1,000 (1)	1,000 (1)	500 (2)	0 (1)	– (0)	0 (1)	– (0)	0 (1)	0 (1)	437 (32)

1,876– 2,375	400 (10)	111 (9)	182 (11)	125 (8)	143 (7)	125 (8)	0 (5)	91 (11)	0 (5)	500 (2)	0 (1)	286 (7)	167 (84)
2,376– 2,875	0 (8)	200 (5)	167 (12)	42 (24)	0 (27)	146 (48)	23 (43)	36 (56)	24 (41)	0 (21)	53 (19)	67 (15)	53 (319)
2,876– 3,375	0 (3)	0 (3)	91 (11)	45 (22)	20 (50)	10 (100)	11 (178)	7 (281)	9 (221)	8 (118)	63 (79)	49 (41)	16 (1,107)
3,376– 3,875	0 (2)	0 (3)	0 (2)	0 (15)	176 (17)	34 (89)	24 (211)	9 (454)	4 (479)	8 (265)	29 (137)	18 (55)	14 (1,729)
3,876– 4,375	0 (1)	0 (1)	0 (2)	167 (6)	91 (11)	80 (25)	16 (62)	25 (237)	16 (246)	36 (192)	0 (90)	43 (23)	26 (896)
4,376– 4,875	– (0)	– (0)	– (0)	0 (3)	0 (4)	0 (6)	0 (24)	32 (62)	27 (73)	16 (62)	33 (30)	100 (10)	26 (274)
4,876– 5,375	– (0)	– (0)	– (0)	– (0)	0 (1)	0 (1)	667 (3)	0 (10)	56 (18)	0 (13)	83 (12)	0 (2)	67 (60)
5,376 or more	– (0)	– (0)	– (0)	– (0)	– (0)	0 (1)	0 (1)	0 (6)	0 (4)	1,000 (1)	0 (4)	– (0)	59 (17)
Unknown	1,000 (1)	– (0)	– (0)	0 (2)	0 (2)	0 (4)	50 (20)	32 (31)	65 (31)	143 (7)	0 (6)	100 (10)	61 (114)
Total	466 (58)	154 (26)	167 (42)	73 (82)	58 (120)	53 (285)	22 (548)	16 (1,148)	13 (1,119)	21 (681)	32 (379)	77 (168)	32 (4,656)

The number in parentheses denotes the number of births.

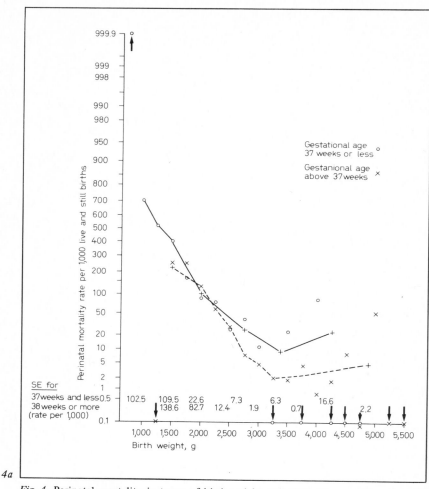

4a

Fig. 4. Perinatal mortality in terms of birth weight, sub-divided by gestational age (all single births) in Göteborg (a) and Palermo (b).

values of the other. The first of what can be termed these 'conditional' relationships is illustrated in figure 4, which shows for single births the way in which perinatal mortality varies with birth weight for the two sections of the population having respectively a gestational age of 37 weeks or less and more than 37 weeks. Ideally, the data should have been sub-divided into more than two groups in terms of gestation, but because of the small numbers of perinatal deaths this could not be done without producing an unduly unstable relationship. On both surveys and for both gestation groups, the mortality-birth weight relationship is

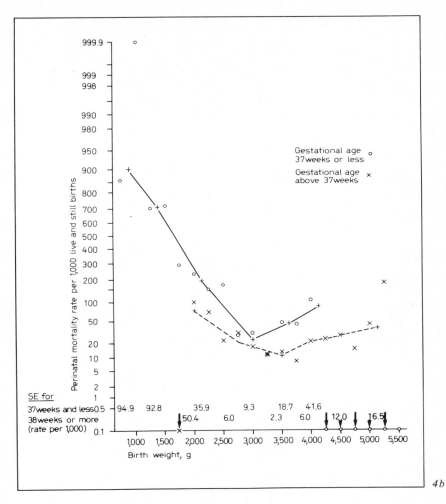

4b

of a similar form to that for all gestational ages. At a given birth weight, mortality in the low gestation group is for the most part consistently higher than in the high gestation groups, although there is some overlap for low weight births at Göteborg. Mortality rates for given birth weight and gestational age group are substantially higher at Palermo than at Göteborg. Indeed, the mortality-birth weight relation for the low gestation group at Göteborg is very similar to that for the high gestation group at Palermo.

Figure 5 shows the relationships between perinatal mortality and gestational

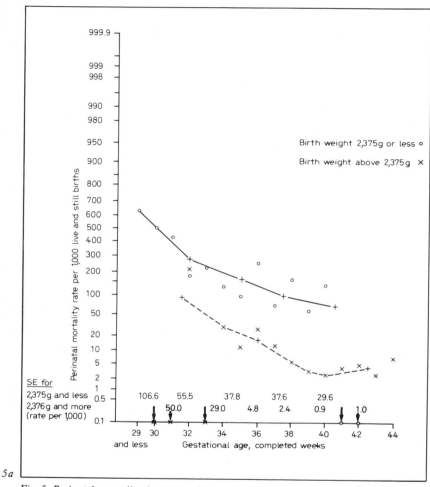

Fig. 5. Perinatal mortality in terms of gestational age, sub-divided by birth weight (all single births) in Göteborg (a) and Palermo (b).

age for single births weighing 2,378 g or less and more than 2,375 g. This cut-off point has been chosen in preference to the more obvious 2,500 g to ameliorate the effects of digit preference. Amongst the low weight births, mortality tends to decrease with increasing gestation and the results for the two surveys are in fairly close agreement over most of the range of gestational age though the missing deaths from Palermo would probably lessen the similarity. Mortality at a given gestational age is markedly lower in the higher birth weight group than in the low birth weight group on both surveys. However, amongst the higher weight

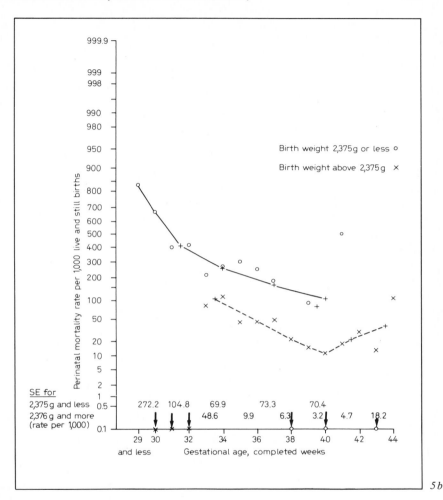

5b

births, the mortality at Palermo is substantially higher than at Göteborg at all gestational ages.

Figures 4 and 5 suggest that birth weight and gestational age are each important in their own right as determinants of mortality, notwithstanding the fact that both qualities are moderately well correlated measures of different aspects of maturity. Further insight into these relationships is given in table I, which shows the perinatal mortality rates corresponding to a detailed sub-division of the data in terms of the two measures jointly. Many of the classes in the off-diagonal positions in the table contain no subjects and the corresponding rates have been left blank. The majority of the observations in both surveys lie in the middle of table I, in the range of birth weight between 2,876 and 4,375 g and of gestational age between 38 and 41 weeks. Many of the more extreme classes contain only a small number of observations and the corresponding mortality rates are subject to a considerable degree of random variation.

Reference to table I a shows that at Göteborg the general form of the mortality-birth weight relationship amongst births of a given gestational age is similar to that in the whole population. This reflects the general trend indicated in figure 4 using a coarse grouping in terms of gestation. When birth weight is fixed, the relation between mortality and gestational age follows the general trend noted in figure 5. Table I b shows that a similar pattern exists at Palermo, although on this survey there is a more pronounced tendency for mortality conditional upon a given gestational age to fall with increasing birth weight, reach a minimum and subsequently to increase as birthweight increases still further. At Göteborg, the perinatal mortality rates within this range were 7 per 1,000 or below, whilst at Palermo the lowest rate was 4 per 1,000 and the highest was 36 per 1,000. If the limits on gestational age are relaxed, mortality rates at Palermo tend to increase markedly as the deviation from the average gestation (40 weeks) becomes larger in either direction, whilst at Göteborg movement in the direction of higher gestation produces only a slight increase. On both surveys, there is a steep increase in mortality between the centre and the top left hand corner of the table. At Palermo, movement in the opposite direction also tends to produce higher mortality rates, but at Göteborg the reported rates for the high birth weight, high gestation births are extremely low. Evidently, the curves for mortality rate against gestational age for a given birth weight are considerably more shallow than those for mortality against birth weight for a given gestational age. This, and other things, suggest that birth weight will be more important than gestational age in explaining variations in mortality levels.[1]

Representative measurements of birth length were obtained at Göteborg and the relation between perinatal mortality and birth length, sub-divided by birth weight, is shown in table II. The pattern of results is similar to that in tables I a and b, high mortality rates being reported for the low weight, small length births. For a given birth weight, we would expect the mortality rate to decrease as we increase birth length from zero, reach a minimum and then to increase for the various birth weight groups of table II. There is some evidence of a decreasing phase in Göteborg from table II (especially in the group 2,376—2,875 g), but

---

[1] It is worth remarking here that a more cohesive pattern would result from plotting contours of equal mortality risk *provided* that these could be made sufficiently smooth. One of us (R.A.H.) is currently developing such a mathematical model.

nowhere near as much as we might have expected to find. This may be partly due to the way birth lengths have been grouped. On the other hand, the increasing phase is very clear. Some further support for the decreasing phase comes from figure 7 where birth weights are split at 2,375 g and aggregated, though the interpretation of this figure is actually equivocal. Note that the difference between the two plots in figure 7 is considerable, indicating the importance of birth weight. Figure 6 shows birth length to be less important, since splitting the data at 445 mm produces more similar plots. There is little doubt that the response lines differ from 2,000 g or so onward, but it is actually the group 446 mm and more which shows the higher mortality rates among the lowest birth weights. This behaviour, which is interesting, is not illogical but is certainly more extreme than that shown by gestational age. Since in addition the range of variation shown by the mortality rate-birth weight plots for given birth length easily exceeds that of the mortality rate-birth length plots for a given birth weight, we must conclude that influence of birth weight is much the stronger, but this is not to say that we can afford to neglect birth length.

IV. Perinatal Mortality, Maturity and Characteristics of the Mother and Child

On the evidence presented above, we have selected birth weight as the most appropriate single predictor of mortality. It is well known that perinatal mortality rates in populations reflect other characteristics of the mother, the infant and the delivery in addition to maturity. The perinatal mortality-birth weight relationship has therefore been examined in terms of some of these other characteristics.

Figure 8 shows that the general pattern of the relationship for single male and female births separately is similar to that for the overall data. At Göteborg, the mortality rates for males in the 1,500–3,000 g birth weight range are higher than for females. In contrast, the Palermo data show no consistent differences in mortality rate between the two sexes. Although differences are not statistically significant with the sample sizes available, it is interesting to note that females show higher mortality rates than males in the highest birth weights at Göteborg, whereas the converse is true in Palermo. The differences between the two sexes in birth weight distribution noted in section III affect the upper part of the range of birth weights only. The result of combining birth weight distribution with the perinatal mortality-birth weight relation produced overall perinatal mortality rates per 1,000 live and still births for singleton males and females of 13.5 and 9.2, respectively, at Göteborg and 36 and 29 respectively at Palermo. The difference in perinatal mortality rates between males and females at Göteborg is significant at the 0.1% level and at Palermo is significant at the 5% level.

Table II. Perinatal mortality in terms of birth weight and birth length: Göteborg. Rate per 1,000 live and still-births

Birth weight, g	Birth length, mm											Total
	≤355	356–385	386–415	416–445	446–475	476–505	506–535	536–565	566–595	≥596	unknown	
≤875	1,000 (13)	1,000 (2)	1,000 (1)	– (0)	– (0)	– (0)	– (0)	– (0)	– (0)	– (0)	1,000 (1)	1,000 (17)
876–1,375	600 (5)	526 (19)	556 (18)	750 (4)	1,000 (2)	– (0)	– (0)	– (0)	– (0)	– (0)	1,000 (2)	600 (50)
1,376–1,875	– (0)	0 (1)	190 (21)	238 (42)	444 (9)	– (0)	– (0)	– (0)	– (0)	– (0)	0 (2)	240 (75)
1,876–2,375	– (0)	– (0)	1,000 (1)	36 (55)	77 (142)	36 (28)	1,000 (1)	– (0)	– (0)	– (0)	200 (5)	73 (232)
2,376–2,875	– (0)	1,000 (1)	– (0)	67 (15)	8 (486)	21 (529)	48 (21)	– (0)	– (0)	– (0)	200 (5)	18 (1,057)
2,876–3,375	– (0)	– (0)	– (0)	– (0)	0 (284)	2 (2,749)	6 (662)	0 (8)	– (0)	– (0)	500 (6)	4 (3,709)
3,376–3,875	– (0)	– (0)	– (0)	– (0)	0 (10)	2 (1,648)	3 (2,601)	26 (151)	0 (2)	– (0)	0 (1)	3 (4,413)
3,876–4,375	– (0)	– (0)	– (0)	– (0)	– (0)	0 (169)	0 (1,467)	7 (401)	143 (7)	– (0)	0 (3)	2 (2,047)

4,376–4,875	5 (391)	— (0)	0 (1)	0 (9)	9 (212)	0 (168)	0 (1)	— (0)	— (0)	— (0)	— (0)	— (0)
4,876–5,375	43 (46)	— (0)	1,000 (1)	143 (7)	0 (28)	0 (10)	— (0)	— (0)	— (0)	— (0)	— (0)	— (0)
5,376 or more	0 (2)	— (0)	— (0)	0 (2)	— (0)	— (0)	— (0)	— (0)	— (0)	— (0)	— (0)	— (0)
Unknown	— (0)	— (0)	— (0)	— (0)	— (0)	— (0)	— (0)	— (0)	— (0)	— (0)	— (0)	— (0)
Total	11 (12,039)	320 (25)	500 (2)	74 (27)	11 (800)	3 (4,930)	4 (5,124)	23 (933)	138 (116)	390 (41)	565 (23)	889 (18)

The number in parentheses denotes the number of births.

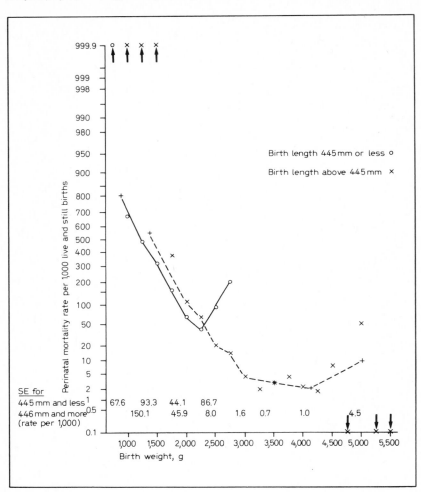

Fig. 6. Perinatal mortality: birth weight relationship in terms of birth length (all single births) in Göteborg.

It is interesting that no significant differences between males and females exist for late neonatal mortality or for mortality between one month and one year.

  The effect of maternal age is illustrated in figure 9 which shows the result of sub-dividing the data for the two surveys in terms of three maternal age groups, below 20 years, 20–34 years and above 34 years. At Göteborg (fig. 9 a), the highest rates were reported for the above 34-year age group and, for birth weights up to about 3,000 g, the lowest rates were reported for the below 20-year age group. For birth weights of above 3,000 g, however, the relative

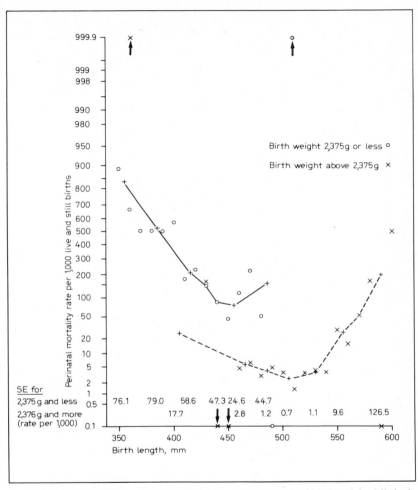

Fig. 7. Perinatal mortality: birth length relationship in terms of birth weight (all single births) in Göteborg.

positions of the below 20-year and 20–34-year maternal age groups are reversed. The results for Palermo (fig. 9 b) show a similar pattern, although the separation between the 20–34-year and above 34-year maternal age groups is more marked.

The perinatal mortality data are summarised in terms of seven maternal age groups in tables III a, b, c which refer respectively to all birth weights, birth weights below 2,501 g and birth weights above 2,500 g. For each entry of table III, both the mortality rate and its standard error are recorded. When all birth weights are considered, the results for both surveys show a tendency for

Table III. Perinatal mortality in terms of place of confinement and maternal age. Rate per 1,000 live and still-births (and SE)

Place of confinement	Maternal age, years							
	19 and under	20–24	25–29	30–34	35–39	40–44	45 and over	all
a) All birth weights								
Göteborg								
West Hospital	11 (7)	15 (3)	12 (2)	10 (3)	37 (11)	63 (30)	0 (–)	15 (2)
East Hospital	15 (6)	8 (2)	12 (2)	16 (4)	10 (6)	0 (–)	0 (–)	11 (1)
Both	14 (5)	11 (2)	12 (2)	13 (3)	23 (6)	29 (14)	0 (–)	13 (1)
Palermo								
University Hospital	16 (16)	37 (12)	24 (9)	71 (17)	70 (23)	151 (53)	333 (272)	49 (7)
Public Hospital A	53 (15)	54 (10)	81 (13)	72 (16)	132 (27)	149 (42)	500 (354)	76 (7)
Public Hospital B	24 (10)	44 (10)	58 (14)	77 (19)	99 (26)	114 (41)	0 (–)	57 (6)
Public Hospitals A or B	22 (22)	5 (5)	43 (14)	65 (24)	173 (44)	86 (58)	0 (–)	52 (9)
Private clinic	12 (6)	12 (3)	10 (2)	17 (4)	20 (6)	43 (19)	142 (132)	14 (2)
Home	29 (9)	11 (3)	15 (4)	13 (5)	25 (9)	34 (17)	0 (–)	16 (2)
All	27 (5)	23 (2)	26 (3)	34 (4)	56 (6)	82 (13)	150 (80)	35 (2)

b) Birth weights below 2,501 g

Göteborg								
West Hospital	115 (63)	178 (38)	231 (44)	154 (58)	368 (111)	333 (157)	—	204 (24)
East Hospital	222 (98)	126 (36)	176 (37)	154 (50)	53 (51)	0 (–)	—	147 (20)
Both	159 (55)	150 (24)	201 (28)	154 (38)	211 (66)	231 (117)	—	174 (15)
Palermo								
University Hospital	250 (217)	250 (97)	0 (–)	291 (93)	333 (136)	666 (274)	1,000 (–)	284 (52)
Public Hospital A	280 (90)	175 (53)	393 (79)	434 (103)	499 (107)	427 (187)	1,000 (–)	340 (37)
Public Hospital B	150 (80)	378 (80)	374 (99)	235 (103)	500 (158)	500 (204)	—	332 (44)
Public Hospitals A or B	—	0 (–)	400 (219)	166 (152)	800 (179)	0 (–)	—	259 (86)
Private clinic	83 (80)	190 (61)	163 (47)	44 (31)	137 (64)	1,000 (–)	—	150 (26)
Home	190 (86)	171 (70)	96 (53)	105 (70)	416 (142)	0 (–)	—	163 (34)
All	190 (43)	220 (30)	229 (32)	193 (34)	365 (51)	444 (96)	1,000 (–)	245 (16)

c) Birth weights above 2,500 g

Göteborg								
West Hospital	0 (–)	5 (2)	3 (1)	5 (2)	14 (7)	18 (18)	0 (–)	5 (1)
East Hospital	3 (4)	2 (1)	5 (1)	8 (3)	7 (5)	0 (–)	0 (–)	4 (1)
Both	3 (2)	3 (1)	4 (1)	6 (1)	11,(4)	8 (8)	0 (1)	4 (1)
Palermo								
University Hospital	0 (–)	20 (9)	25 (10)	45 (15)	42 (19)	115 (49)	0 (–)	31 (6)
Public Hospital A	25 (11)	40 (9)	51 (11)	37 (12)	73 (22)	121 (40)	0 (–)	54 (6)
Public Hospital B	13 (8)	12 (6)	28 (10)	63 (18)	66 (23)	72 (35)	0 (–)	30 (5)
Public Hospitals A or B	22 (22)	5 (5)	35 (13)	60 (24)	128 (40)	100 (67)	0 (–)	45 (8)
Private clinic	9 (5)	6 (2)	4 (2)	15 (4)	14 (5)	9 (9)	142 (132)	8 (1)
Home	18 (7)	6 (3)	11 (4)	11 (4)	12 (6)	36 (18)	0 (–)	11 (2)
All	14 (3)	12 (2)	16 (2)	23 (3)	30 (5)	61 (12)	55 (54)	19 (1)

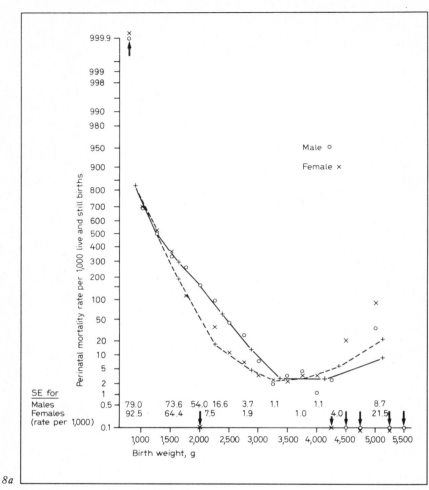

8a

Fig. 8. Perinatal mortality: birth weight relationship in terms of sex (all single births) in Göteborg (a) and Palermo (b).

mortality to decrease initially with increasing maternal age, reaching a minimum in the 20–24-year age group and subsequently to increase as maternal age increases still further. This latter trend is very much more pronounced at Palermo than at Göteborg and the average rate at Palermo is almost three times as high as that at Göteborg in the 40–44 year age group, in comparison with about twice as high in the 19-year and under and 20–24-year age groups. When the data are sub-divided in terms of place of confinement, the same general trends apply, although because of smaller numbers of cases the individual rates are subject to a

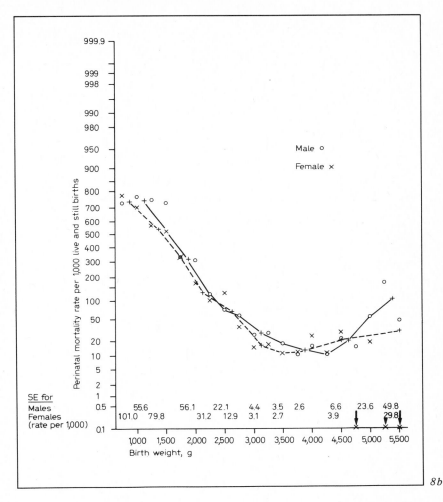

8b

greater degree of random variation. It is interesting that at Palermo the rates for births taking place at home or in private clinics are consistently lower than those for births taking place in hospital for all maternal age groups. The mortality rates for the low weight births are less closely related to maternal age than the overall data. It is interesting that in the 25–34-year age groups, mortality rates in the two surveys are similar, although Göteborg is at a marked advantage for the lower maternal ages. The higher birth weight groups (table IIIc) exhibit the same general trends as the data for all birth weights. At Göteborg, there is almost a

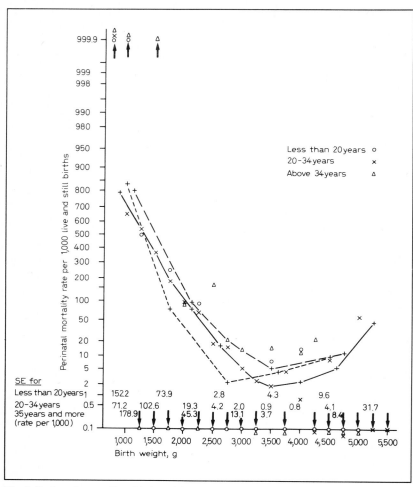

9a

Fig. 9. Perinatal mortality: birth weight relationship in terms of maternal age (all single births) in Göteborg (a) and Palermo (b).

fourfold increase between perinatal mortality rates in the under 20-year and over 34-year maternal age groups. The differences in mortality rates between the various places of confinement at Palermo persist in both birth weight classes and throughout the range of maternal ages.[2]

The distribution of maternal age on the two surveys is summarised in

[2] It should be pointed out that 12% of perinatal deaths in Palermo have unknown weights. Many might be included in table III b if they were known, thus increasing mortality rates, especially in the extreme age groups.

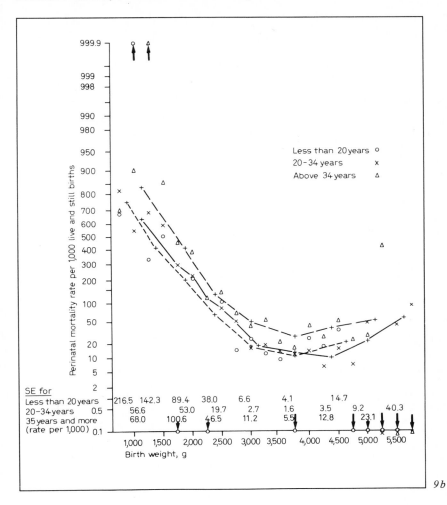

9b

table IV. The proportion of births at the two extremes of the maternal age distribution is considerably higher at Palermo than at Göteborg. Mothers of less than 19 years of age at Public Hospital B (where the overall mortality rate is very high) are represented to a much greater extent than in the Palermo survey generally, whereas the reverse applies for private clinics and the University Hospital. It is clear from table III that such differences in maternal age can account for only part of the variations in mortality rates between the various places of confinement at Palermo or indeed between the two surveys.

Table IV. Maternal age in terms of place of confinement, all birth weights included. Rate per 1,000 live and still-births

Place of confinement	Maternal age, years							
	19 and under	20–24	25–29	30–34	35–39	40–44	45 and over	all
Göteborg								
West Hospital	47	295	403	188	54	11	2	1,000
East Hospital	59	358	385	172	44	11	1	1,000
Both	53	330	393	163	49	11	1	1,000
Palermo								
University Hospital	61	262	278	221	126	45	2	1,000
Public Hospital A	139	302	257	157	96	44	1	1,000
Public Hospital B	182	313	203	153	97	45	2	1,000
Public Hospitals A or B	71	282	319	168	119	36	1	1,000
Private clinic	62	273	334	202	102	23	1	1,000
Home	118	287	262	189	104	35	1	1,000
All	99	284	287	188	104	33	1	1,000

The distribution of perinatal mortality in terms of birth weight and parity is illustrated in figure 10, in which parity is sub-divided in terms of three classes: 0, 1–2, and 3 or more. At Palermo, the assessment of parity is based upon the number of previous pregnancies proceeding beyond 28 weeks of gestation, the generally accepted definition. At Göteborg, on the other hand, the information available is summarised in terms of the number of previous live and stillbirths, multiple pregnancies being counted twice (or more often). This difference in definition only affects the small proportion of mothers with previous multiple pregnancies. The results on the two surveys show a very similar pattern, in that mortality rates for the parity 3 or more births are substantially higher than the remainder. Differences between parity 0 and parity 1 and 2 are small at Göteborg, but at Palermo the rates for the former are consistently higher than for the latter for birth weights up to about 3,000 g.

The data are also summarised in a different way in tables Va, b and c, which refer respectively to all birth weights and to births weighing below 2,501 g and above 2,500 g. On both surveys, mortality rates fall with increasing parity, reach a minimum at parity 2 and subsequently increase very sharply, the pattern being particularly marked at Palermo. A similar pattern applies for each place of confinement, although the minimum is reached for parity 1 rather than for parity 2 in some cases. The large fall in mortality rate between parity 0 and parity 2 for confinements taking place at home at Palermo is particularly interesting, since the rate of 6 per 1,000 for parity 2 for this place of confinement is one of the lowest figures quoted in table V for either survey. Reference to tables Vb and c show that the same general pattern of variation of mortality with parity persists at Göteborg when low weight and higher weight births are considered separately, although there is no consistent difference between parity 0 and parity 1. At Palermo, on the other hand, the mortality rates amongst the higher weight births are very similar for parity 0, 1 and 2, whilst the low weight births have a clearly defined minimum for mortality at parity 1 and 2.

Table VI shows the distribution of parity in the various places of confinement on the two surveys. At Göteborg, more than half the births were classed as parity 0, compared with about 37% at Palermo. On the other hand, almost 20% of the Palermo births were parity 3 or more, in comparison with less than 5% at Göteborg. These differences can only, however, account for a small part of the variations in mortality rate between the two surveys. At Palermo, it is interesting that less than 20% of the deliveries taking place at home were parity 0, whilst as many as 37% were parity 3 or more. In the private clinics, however, some 43% of the deliveries were parity 0 and only about 10% were parity 3 or more.

It is appropriate to add a word of caution in interpretation relative to the distribution of infants over the various places of confinement in Palermo for the total survey. This is different from that produced by the 'edited standard record sample', together with mortality rates.

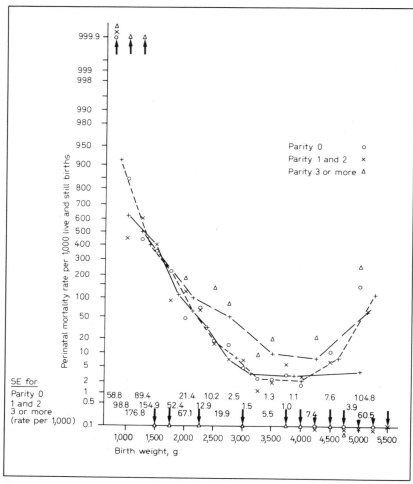

10a

Fig. 10. Perinatal mortality: birth weight relationship in terms of parity (all single births) in Göteborg (a) and Palermo (b).

When considered separately, both maternal age and parity are associated with perinatal mortality. However, because in any particular family both parity and maternal age must inevitably increase in step, the two factors are closely correlated in a population. For this reason, an analysis has been carried out of the relation between maternal age and parity jointly and perinatal mortality and the results are summarised in tables VIIa and b, which refer respectively to Göteborg and Palermo. For a given maternal age with substantial numbers of births of more than one parity, mortality tends to decrease between parity 0 and

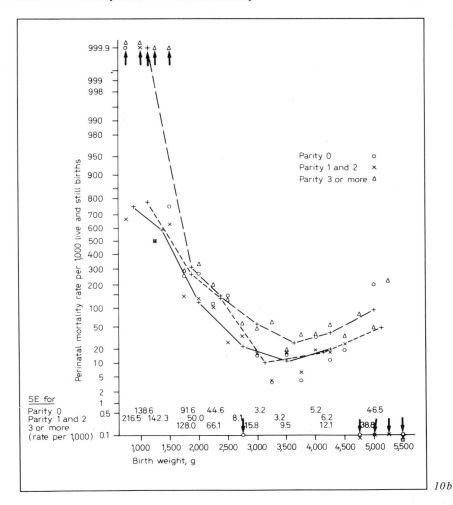

10b

parity 1, to reach a minimum at parity 1 or parity 2 and subsequently to increase again as parity increases still further. The trends are more consistent at Göteborg than at Palermo, particularly in the over 30-year age groups. For a given parity, there is a general tendency for mortality first to fall and subsequently to rise as maternal age increases. The maternal age corresponding to the minimum mortality tends to increase with increasing parity.

The joint distribution of maternal age and parity in the two populations is shown in tables VIIIa and b. The proportion of high parity, high maternal age

Table V. Perinatal mortality in terms of place of confinement and parity. Rate per 1,000 live and still-births (and SE)

Place of confinement	Parity							
	0	1	2	3	4	5	6+	all
a) All birth weights								
Göteborg								
West Hospital	14 (2)	17 (3)	6 (3)	30 (12)	18 (18)	38 (37)	0 (–)	15 (2)
East Hospital	13 (2)	8 (2)	4 (2)	26 (11)	28 (19)	65 (44)	0 (–)	11 (1)
Both	14 (1)	12 (2)	5 (2)	28 (8)	24 (13)	53 (30)	0 (–)	13 (1)
Palermo (edited standard records)								
University Hospital	28 (12)	33 (13)	72 (35)	64 (44)	71 (69)	111 (105)	362 (145)	48 (10)
Public Hospital A	43 (16)	31 (13)	0 (–)	38 (27)	95 (64)	0 (–)	113 (48)	38 (8)
Public Hospital B	57 (14)	68 (21)	56 (22)	94 (37)	110 (52)	58 (57)	118 (37)	70 (10)
Public Hospitals A or B	–	–	–	–	–	–	–	–
Private clinic	15 (4)	13 (4)	17 (8)	48 (19)	80 (38)	0 (–)	184 (70)	20 (3)
Home	36 (15)	10 (23)	6 (6)	43 (19)	0 (–)	42 (29)	54 (26)	23 (5)
All	28 (4)	23 (4)	22 (6)	54 (12)	52 (15)	34 (17)	116 (22)	33 (3)

b) Birth weights less than 2,501 g

Göteborg							
West Hospital	176 (30)	288 (53)	111 (60)	364 (145)	0 (–)	0 (–)	500 (356)	204 (24)
East Hospital	179 (29)	109 (32)	86 (47)	154 (100)	200 (179)	0 (–)	0 (–)	147 (20)
Both	178 (21)	188 (30)	97 (37)	250 (88)	100 (95)	0 (–)	333 (272)	174 (15)

Palermo (edited standard records)							
University Hospital	307 (128)	142 (130)	250 (153)	–	–	1,000 (–)	–	275 (83)
Public Hospital A	500 (144)	272 (95)	333 (272)	0 (–)	600 (219)	0 (–)	333 (192)	333 (64)
Public Hospital B	384 (95)	428 (187)	444 (166)	500 (158)	1,000 (–)	–	1,000 (–)	454 (67)
Public Hospitals A or B	–	–	–	–	–	–	–	–
Private clinic	138 (57)	208 (75)	76 (73)	500 (353)	–	0 (–)	1,000 (–)	175 (42)
Home	222 (139)	–	125 (171)	333 (192)	0 (–)	0 (–)	500 (250)	166 (57)
All	262 (45)	168 (45)	170 (63)	363 (103)	544 (150)	90 (86)	582 (142)	246 (29)

c) Birth weights above 2,500 g

Göteborg							
West Hospital	4 (1)	5 (2)	2 (2)	11 (7)	20 (19)	0 (–)	0 (–)	5 (1)
East Hospital	4 (1)	4 (1)	0 (–)	17 (10)	15 (15)	0 (–)	123 (88)	4 (1)
Both	4 (1)	4 (1)	1 (1)	13 (6)	17 (12)	0 (–)	53 (36)	4 (1)

Palermo (edited standard records)							
University Hospital	10 (7)	14 (10)	24 (24)	32 (32)	0 (–)	0 (–)	166 (135)	16 (6)
Public Hospital A	19 (11)	29 (14)	0 (–)	27 (27)	45 (46)	0 (–)	64 (35)	23 (7)
Public Hospital B	26 (11)	45 (18)	28 (16)	39 (27)	33 (33)	71 (69)	96 (38)	39 (7)
Public Hospitals A or B	–	–	–	–	–	–	–	–
Private clinic	12 (3)	7 (3)	14 (7)	41 (18)	65 (36)	0 (–)	103 (56)	14 (3)
Home	19 (11)	9 (7)	5 (5)	18 (13)	12 (12)	22 (22)	48 (24)	16 (4)
All	12 (3)	13 (3)	13 (5)	39 (10)	26 (12)	28 (16)	83 (20)	19 (2)

Table VI. Parity in terms of place of confinement. Rate per 1,000 live and still-births

Place of confinement	Parity							
	0	1	2	3	4	5	6 +	all
Göteborg								
West Hospital	510	315	119	36	10	5	4	1,000
East Hospital	511	339	104	28	11	5	2	1,000
Both	511	328	111	32	10	5	3	1,000
Palermo (edited standard records)								
University Hospital	432	311	117	66	29	19	23	1,000
Public Hospital A	312	304	138	102	41	29	69	1,000
Public Hospital B	388	203	150	88	50	23	94	1,000
Public Hospitals A or B	–	–	–	–	–	–	–	–
Private clinic	435	330	128	56	22	13	12	1,000
Home	193	232	195	133	102	55	87	1,000
All	371	289	143	80	44	24	45	1,000

births at Palermo is substantially greater than at Göteborg. Nevertheless, comparison of tables VIIa and b shows that for all combinations of parity and maternal age, mortality at Palermo is consistently higher than at Göteborg. The excess in overall mortality at Palermo can only be attributed in part to the adverse parity-maternal age distribution.

At Palermo, the occupation of the husband (or head of the mother's household if not the husband) was recorded on the standard records and the resulting information was classified in terms of 'social class' on the basis of the system used by the Registrar General of England and Wales (General Register Office, 1966). Perinatal mortality has been summarised in terms of social classes 1–2 (professional and managerial), 3 (other 'white collar' and skilled manual), 4–5 (semi-skilled and unskilled manual). Occupations such as students and members of the armed forces which do not conform to the general system have been classified separately as category 0. The results obtained are summarised in tables IX and X, which refer to the joint classification of social class with maternal age and parity, respectively. When social class is considered in isolation, perinatal mortality increases as social class decreases. The same general trend holds for maternal ages up to 24 years and for parity 0 births. However, for higher maternal ages and parities there is no consistent pattern, probably because of the relatively small numbers of deliveries in social classes 1–2 and 4–5. When the data are sub-divided in terms of birth weight, the tendency for mortality to increase with decreasing social class is present in both the below 2,501-gram and above 2,500-gram groups. The missing numbers of observations should be mentioned finally.

V. Perinatal Mortality and Complications of Pregnancy and Delivery

On the Göteborg survey, a prospective record was made for clinical purposes of various aspects of the obstetric history, including complications of pregnancy, which have been classified in terms of toxaemia, ante-partum haemorrhage, vaginal bleeding before the 28th week of gestation and other illnesses. At Palermo, on the other hand, a similar set of information was collected retrospectively as part of the standard records. The prevalence of the selected complications at the various places of confinement on the two surveys is summarised in table XI and the perinatal mortality rates for the various classes are shown in table XII. Because of the relatively low prevalence of the various complications, analysis in terms of birth weight was not worthwhile.

In the classification of toxaemia of pregnancy the following definitions were used: mild – systolic pressure 140–150 mm Hg; moderate – systolic pressure 150–160 mm Hg; severe – systolic pressure above 160 mm Hg or below 140 mm Hg plus oedema and proteinuria. The reported rates of toxaemia, and

Table VII. Perinatal mortality in terms of maternal age and parity, all birth weights included. Rate per 1,000 live and still-births (and SE)

Parity	Maternal age, years							
	19 and under	20–24	25–29	30–34	35–39	40–44	45 and over	all
a) Göteborg								
0	13 (5)	12 (2)	13 (2)	22 (6)	30 (17)	0 (–)	– (–)	13 (1)
1	23 (22)	8 (3)	12 (2)	11 (4)	29 (13)	37 (36)	0 (–)	12 (2)
2	0 (–)	7 (7)	8 (4)	2 (2)	6 (6)	0 (–)	0 (–)	5 (2)
3	0 (–)	77 (74)	18 (12)	26 (12)	34 (19)	50 (49)	0 (–)	28 (8)
4	– (–)	0 (–)	38 (37)	0 (–)	25 (25)	62 (60)	– (–)	23 (13)
5	– (–)	– (–)	0 (–)	0 (–)	0 (–)	0 (–)	0 (–)	0 (–)
6 or more	– (–)	0 (–)	0 (–)	166 (152)	48 (46)	111 (105)	0 (–)	73 (41)
All	14 (5)	11 (2)	12 (2)	13 (2)	23 (6)	29 (14)	0 (–)	13 (1)
b) Palermo (edited standard records)								
0	32 (9)	24 (6)	24 (7)	44 (16)	47 (33)	0 (–)	–	28 (4)
1	16 (11)	12 (5)	14 (5)	44 (14)	68 (25)	71 (69)	–	23 (4)
2	37 (36)	24 (12)	15 (9)	25 (11)	10 (10)	76 (74)	0 (–)	21 (6)
3	250 (217)	33 (23)	65 (24)	29 (17)	48 (23)	94 (6)	1,000 (–)	52 (11)
4		41 (40)	40 (28)	45 (26)	115 (49)	0 (–)	0 (–)	52 (15)
5		0 (–)	0 (–)	76 (42)	0 (–)	142 (132)	0 (–)	34 (17)
6 or more		0 (–)	0 (–)	114 (41)	152 (42)	194 (66)	0 (–)	116 (226)
All	27 (7)	23 (4)	26 (4)	34 (6)	56 (11)	82 (26)	150 (146)	35 (3)

Table VIII. Maternal age and parity. Rate per 1,000 live and still-births

Parity	Maternal age, years							all
	19 and under	20–24	25–29	30–34	35–39	40–44	45 and over	
a) Göteborg								
0	49	229	177	45	8	2	0	509
1	3	88	158	62	14	2	0	328
2	0	11	45	38	13	3	0	111
3	0	1	9	13	7	2	0	32
4	0	0	2	4	3	1	0	10
5	0	0	1	1	2	0	0	4
6 or more	0	0	0	0	2	1	1	3
All	53	330	393	163	49	11	1	1,000
b) Palermo (edited standard records)								
0	78	148	94	37	9	3	0	371
1	26	84	104	48	21	3	0	289
2	5	33	39	41	21	2	0	143
3	0	12	22	21	17	4	0	81
4	0	5	10	14	9	4	0	43
5	0	2	5	8	7	1	0	24
6 or more	0	0	6	11	14	8	1	43
All	112	287	285	184	101	26	1	1,000

Table IX. Perinatal mortality in terms of maternal age and social class in Palermo (edited standard records), all birth weights included. Rate per 1,000 live and still-births (and SE)

Maternal age, years	Social class				
	1−2	3	4−5	0	all
19 and under	0 (−)	24 (9)	43 (21)	66 (29)	27 (5)
20−24	0 (−)	18 (5)	24 (10)	39 (16)	23 (2)
25−29	12 (7)	27 (6)	15 (9)	24 (14)	26 (3)
30−34	39 (16)	36 (9)	80 (22)	41 (20)	34 (4)
35−39	72 (35)	62 (15)	43 (19)	106 (41)	56 (6)
40−44	0 (−)	74 (36)	108 (51)	142 (66)	82 (13)
45 and over	1,000 (−)	−	0 (−)	−	150 (80)
All	21 (6)	30 (3)	40 (7)	50 (9)	35 (2)

Table X. Perinatal mortality in terms of parity and social class in Palermo (edited standard records), all birth weights included. Rate per 1,000 live and still-births (and SE)

Parity	Social class				
	1−2	3	4−5	0	all
0	6 (5)	27 (5)	40 (13)	46 (16)	28 (4)
1	27 (11)	17 (5)	38 (13)	25 (14)	23 (4)
2	12 (12)	29 (8)	9 (9)	16 (16)	22 (6)
3	45 (44)	52 (15)	44 (22)	81 (35)	54 (12)
4	222 (139)	56 (22)	17 (17)	55 (38)	52 (15)
5	333 (272)	34 (24)	30 (30)	0 (−)	34 (17)
6 +	0 (−)	108 (37)	70 (28)	145 (26)	116 (22)
All	20 (6)	29 (3)	41 (7)	50 (9)	33 (3)

particularly the mild form, are very considerably higher at Göteborg than at Palermo. Clearly, the difference is so large that reporting errors seem to be involved. It seems very likely that the more intensive and systematic regime of antenatal care at Göteborg has tended to bring to light many more mild symptoms than are noted at Palermo. This hypothesis is consistent with the fact that the reported prevalence of mild toxaemia is more than twice as high at the East Hospital than at the West Hospital. At Palermo, the reported prevalence of toxaemia is very low for mothers delivered in private clinics, at home and in Public Hospital A and is considerably higher for the University Hospital and Public Hospital B. The perinatal mortality rates for the various grades of toxaemia show no consistent pattern. At Göteborg, mortality amongst the mothers

Table XI. Place of confinement and complications of pregnancy. Rate per 1,000 live and still-births

Place of confinement	Toxaemia				Ante-partum haemorrhage		Vaginal bleeding before 28th week		Other illness	
	none	mild	moderate	severe	no	yes	no	yes	no	yes
Göteborg										
West Hospital	902	73	20	5	984	16	994	6	840	160
East Hospital	820	161	16	3	968	32	979	21	819	181
Both	857	121	18	4	975	25	985	15	826	174
Palermo (edited standard records)										
University Hospital	931	31	14	21	970	29	882	117	961	38
Public Hospital A	969	11	5	13	961	38	938	61	923	76
Public Hospital B	911	51	14	21	971	28	922	77	907	92
Private clinic	988	7	0	2	985	14	902	97	814	185
Home	985	10	1	2	974	25	926	73	792	207
All	968	17	5	8	977	22	911	88	851	148

Table XII. Perinatal mortality in terms of place of confinement and complications of pregnancy. Rate per 1,000 live and still-births

Place of confinement	Toxaemia				Ante-partum haemorrhage		Vaginal bleeding before 28th week		Other illness	
	none	mild	moderate	severe	no	yes	no	yes	no	yes
Göteborg										
West Hospital	14	11	27	214	14	34	15	29	12	19
East Hospital	13	3	18	59	11	33	11	36	11	18
Both	13	5	23	155	13	33	13	34	12	18
Palermo (edited standard records)										
University Hospital	38	0	285	0	31	0	37	54	34	166
Public Hospital A	38	166	0	427	38	200	44	62	44	50
Public Hospital B	77	52	181	0	65	428	67	185	76	58
Private clinic	16	352	0	0	18	93	18	32	19	21
Home	15	222	1,000	0	17	90	19	15	20	16
All	30	129	208	72	30	164	30	54	34	29

with mild toxaemia is considerably lower than for mothers without any of the symptoms of toxaemia. Indeed, the perinatal mortality rate amongst infants born to mothers with mild toxaemia at the East Hospital was only 3 per 1,000, in comparison with 11 per 1,000 at the West Hospital (where the proportion of such cases was very much lower) and both figures are lower than the rates of 13–14 per 1,000 for cases where no symptoms of toxaemia were reported. The close agreement in the mortality rates associated with mothers without toxaemia at the two Göteborg hospitals is interesting. These results are open to several possible interpretations. For example, the risk to infants of mothers with mild toxaemia may really be lower than that associated with mothers without toxaemia. Alternatively, the additional antenatal and other care given to mothers identified as having mild toxaemia is effective in reducing the risk of perinatal death below the level prevailing in the population as a whole. At Göteborg, the perinatal mortality rate associated with moderate toxaemia is higher than that amongst infants born to mothers without toxaemia, but substantially below that associated with the small proportion of mothers with severe toxaemia. At Palermo, the perinatal mortality associated with toxaemia is substantially greater than the average. When all places of confinement are considered together, the mortality associated with moderate toxaemia is higher than that associated either with the mild or the severe forms of the condition. For a given grade of toxaemia, mortality is relatively high for mothers delivered at home, in private nursing homes or in Public Hospital A, where the proportion of mothers assessed as having toxaemia are relatively low.

The proportions of mothers with ante-partum haemorrhage (APH) on both surveys and all places of confinement are low and amount on average to about 1 in 40. It is interesting that the rate reported at the East Hospital at Göteborg is twice as high as at the West Hospital. At Palermo, the highest prevalence of APH was reported for mothers delivered at Public Hospital A and the lowest in the private clinics. Perinatal mortality amongst infants delivered to mothers with APH is on average 2–3 times higher at Göteborg and 4–6 times higher at Palermo than amongst the remainder of the population.

The proportion of mothers who reported vaginal bleeding before the 28th week of gestation was higher at Palermo than at Göteborg. The prevalence at the East Hospital at Göteborg was again higher than at the West Hospital, whereas the extent of the variation between different places of confinement at Palermo was comparatively small. Perinatal mortality was generally higher amongst infants delivered to mothers with this symptom, the relative difference being higher at Göteborg than at Palermo.

A substantial minority of mothers experienced other illnesses during the pregnancy, the average rate being about 175 per 1,000 live and still births at Göteborg and about 150 at Palermo. The pattern of results in the two hospitals at Göteborg was very similar, but at Palermo the prevalence of other illnesses

Table XIII. Place of confinement and method of delivery. Rate per 1,000 live and still-births

Place of confinement	Method of delivery						
	normal	forceps	el. Caes.	em. Caes.	breech	other	all
Göteborg							
West Hospital	755	80	− 52 −		28	85	1,000
East Hospital	796	45	− 65 −		27	67	1,000
Both	777	61	− 59 −		28	75	1,000
Palermo (edited standard records)							
University Hospital	690	70	70	57	38	72	1,000
Public Hospital A	743	65	63	51	42	34	1,000
Public Hospital B	814	70	25	47	38	2	1,000
Private clinic	756	106	55	44	20	15	1,000
Home	928	46	0	0	17	6	1,000
All	788	81	43	38	27	20	1,000

was relatively high for births at home and in private clinics. At Göteborg, the mortality rate associated with other illness was about 50% higher than in the remainder of the population, but at Palermo there was no persistent trend.

In summary, the results suggest that the information concerning complications of pregnancy was questionable in some respects. At Göteborg, the fact that the reported prevalence of toxaemia, of APH and of vaginal bleeding was more than twice as high at the East Hospital than at the West Hospital suggests that different conventions were applied in the assessment and recording of symptoms. The sources of information in the different places of confinement at Palermo were more diverse and this raises the possibility of differing standards. However, apart from mild toxaemia at Göteborg, the results in general reveal a positive association between each of the complications of pregnancy and perinatal mortality.

On each survey a record was made of the method of delivery and each delivery was classified as forceps, vacuum, breech, Caesarian and other intervention, as summarised in table XIII. At Palermo, a distinction was made between elective and emergency Caesarian sections. The average proportions of forceps or vacuum deliveries were comparable on both surveys, but there were some variations between different places of confinement on the same survey. Thus, at Göteborg the use of vacuum extraction was twice as common at the West Hospital than at the East Hospital. At Palermo, the proportion of forceps deliveries was relatively high in the private clinics and relatively low amongst the home deliveries. However, perinatal mortality rates show no consistent differences between forceps deliveries and deliveries which were without complication.

The Caesarian section rate was on average greater at Palermo than at Göteborg, with a level of about 1 in 10 at the latter. At Palermo, the proportions of elective and emergency Caesarian operations are approximately equal and, apart from the home confinements, the rates reported in the hospitals and the private clinics are in fairly close agreement. At Göteborg, the perinatal mortality rate associated with Caesarian section was on average three times that reported for deliveries that were without complication, whilst the rate for the West Hospital was almost twice as high as at the East Hospital. At Palermo, mortality associated with elective Caesarian deliveries was very low. On the other hand, emergency Caesarian operations at the hospitals resulted in a relatively high mortality level. However, for the deliveries taking place in private clinics, the perinatal mortality rate was only half that for the deliveries without complication.

Breech deliveries amounted to about 3% of the total at Göteborg and a slightly higher proportion at Palermo. There was no appreciable difference between the proportions of such deliveries at the two hospitals at Göteborg, but the associated perinatal mortality was higher at the West Hospital. The proportions of breech deliveries at the three Palermo hospitals were also very similar, but mortality at Public Hospital A was substantially lower than at the University Hospital and at Public Hospital B was substantially higher.

Other complications of delivery were associated with about 7.5% of cases at Göteborg and a somewhat lower proportion at Palermo. The overall prevalences of this category on both surveys were similar, but there were considerable variations between the places of confinement at Palermo. The perinatal mortality rates associated with other complications was more than 5 times as high as that for uncomplicated deliveries at Göteborg, but less than twice as high at Palermo.

VI. Comment

The purpose of this paper is to identify characteristics of the mother, the infant, the pregnancy and the delivery which are associated with perinatal mortality. Although analyses of this kind can never prove relationships found to be causal, the results should provide useful pointers to courses of action which may be expected to reduce the risk of perinatal death. Given such information, the way is then open to the development of policies for the delivery of maternity care which will be both effective and efficient.

As anticipated, perinatal mortality varies very widely in terms of each of the indices of maturity. A similar pattern was observed for each index, with mortality falling very sharply from a level of virtually 100% as maturity increases from the lowest observed level, reaching a minimum at the median of the distribution of maturity and subsequently increasing as maturity increases still further. The extent of this latter increase is considerably greater for birth length than for birth weight, but rather less marked for gestational age. When birth weight and gestational age are considered jointly, for a given birth weight mortality increases as gestation decreases. On the other hand, for given gestational age, mortality increases as birth weight decreases. On this basis, birth weight appears to be more closely associated with mortality than gestation. This remark applies with even greater force to birth length and it is clear that gestational age and birth length alone contribute little information about perinatal mortality in addition to that provided by birth weight.

As expected, the overall perinatal mortality rates for males were significantly higher than those for females on both surveys. At Palermo, this difference was associated almost entirely with variations in birth weight distribution and the perinatal mortality-birth weight relation was very similar for the two sexes. At Göteborg, on the other hand, perinatal mortality in the range of birth weights between 1,500 and 3,000 g was consistently higher for males than for females. These results suggest that the extent of the differences between males and females may be associated with the overall level of perinatal mortality in the population. When the results of the two surveys were analysed in terms of maternal age and parity, both separately and jointly, the pattern revealed was of initially decreasing mortality as either factor increases from the lowest levels, followed by a subsequent increase as the higher values are reached. At Palermo, where differences in social class were assessed, mortality increased with decreasing general well-being, as revealed by the occupation of the head of household. These trends are all consistent with the results of surveys carried out in many parts of the world. Apart from mild toxaemia, complications of pregnancy were associated with raised levels of perinatal mortality. A similar remark applies to Caesarian sections, breech deliveries and other complications of delivery except the use of forceps, or vacuum extraction.

When the two surveys are compared, perinatal mortality rates were consistently higher at Palermo than at Göteborg in virtually all categories (table XIV). In terms of maturity, the mortality rates were most similar in the lowest categories, and the relative advantage enjoyed by Göteborg was most pronounced for the categories in the central part of the distribution. Although the Palermo mothers are at a clear disadvantage in terms of parity and maternal age, this difference probably only accounts for a small percentage of the difference in mortality rates.

In terms of the variation between different places of confinement within the same survey, the excess of perinatal mortality at the West Hospital over the East Hospital at Göteborg requires further investigation into the precise case-mix. The analysis suggests that this difference is concentrated largely upon complicated deliveries (other than forceps or vacuum extraction). There is also a suggestion

Table XIV. Perinatal mortality in terms of place of confinement and method of delivery. Rate per 1,000 live and still-births

Place of confinement	Method of delivery					
	normal	forceps	el. Caes.	em. Caes.	breech	other
Göteborg						
West Hospital	8	7	— 31 —		82	47
East Hospital	7	7	— 18 —		55	44
Both	8	7	— 23 —		68	45
Palermo (edited standard records)						
University Hospital	33	30	0	111	221	0
Public Hospital A	51	0	0	74	45	55
Public Hospital B	54	115	0	227	321	0
Private clinic	16	20	8	10	132	93
Home	19	25	—	—	0	0
All	27	32	4	74	155	45

of a difference between the hospitals in terms of antenatal care. A similar set of circumstances may also account for part of the excess of perinatal mortality for deliveries at Public Hospital B at Palermo. There were also large differences between the maternal age and parity distributions between the hospitals, the private clinics and the home confinements at Palermo. However, the overall differences between places of confinement are present within all the categories which were examined. This suggests that case-mix is unlikely to provide a complete explanation and that the results do reflect, at least to some extent, real differences in hazard between the samples having their confinement at various places in Palermo.

Summary

This section presents an analysis of perinatal mortality in terms of birth weight, gestational age and birth length. It is shown that when account is taken of birth weight, gestational age provides little further explanation of differences in mortality and birth length virtually no additional information. The perinatal mortality-birth weight relation is then assessed in terms of parity and maternal age. When these factors are considered both singly and jointly, perinatal mortality tends to decrease initially and subsequently to increase as either moves from the bottom to the top of the range of variation. There were no consistent differences in the perinatal mortality-birth weight relationship in terms of the sex of the child, but largely as a result of differences in birth weight distribution mortality amongst males was significantly higher than amongst females. Mortality rates were also analysed in terms of complications of pregnancy and delivery. It is shown that the differences in overall mortality rates between Göteborg and Palermo persist for all categories considered in this analysis. However, virtually the whole of the variation between the two hospitals at Göteborg and part of the variation between the different places of confinement at Palermo can be accounted for by differences in the characteristics of the mother, the child, the pregnancy or the delivery.

References

General Register Office: Classification of occupations (HMSO, London 1966).

Fryer, J.G.: The relationship between the birth weight of an infant and its probability of survival (submitted for publication and personal commun., 1976).

Prof. *J.R. Ashford,* MA, PhD, FBCS, Head, Department of Mathematical Statistics and Operational Research, University of Exeter, Streatham Court, Rennes Drive, *Exeter EX4 4PU* (England)

Monogr. Paediat., vol. 9, pp. 165–192 (Karger, Basel 1977)

Clinical Evaluation of Similarities and Dissimilarities between the Two City Surveys

P. Karlberg and A. Priolisi

Department of Pediatrics, University of Göteborg, Göteborg and Child Health Institute, University of Palermo, Palermo

Introduction

The aim of this section is a clinical evaluation of similarities and dissimilarities found in the analysis of perinatal data obtained from Göteborg and Palermo. Focus has been on the possibility of estimating the priorities for the improvement of the perinatal care or, better expressed, to reduce the hazard of passing through 'the valley of the shadow of birth' (1). Since increased knowledge of biological phenomena and mechanisms improves clinical care, these factors will also be taken into consideration.

The material consists of information from, and analysis of, 12,271 births in Göteborg and 13,188 births in Palermo, with 190 and 674 deaths up to 1 year after birth, respectively, representing the total birth population reported on in the previous sections.

The perinatal mortality rate of the two cities is quite different, Göteborg 13 and Palermo 35 per 1,000 births (section I), as was expected when the cities were chosen.

When the late neonatal deaths are included — deaths up to 28 days after birth — the difference is even larger: Göteborg 14 and Palermo 47 (i.e. a 3-times difference).

The periods studied, Göteborg 1972 and 1973 (2 years), and Palermo 1971/72 (11 months), form a representative part of the perinatal mortality pattern during the last five decades in each of the two cities (fig. 1).

The perinatal care system is different in the two cities. In Göteborg, perinatal care is organized homogeneously with delivery only taking place in either of two maternity hospitals (3,000 deliveries per year). There is a neonatal unit in each and only one Department of Pediatrics in the city with full responsibility for care of all the newborn infants. These include infants with an uneventful course as well as those showing disturbances or anomalies. In Palermo, perinatal

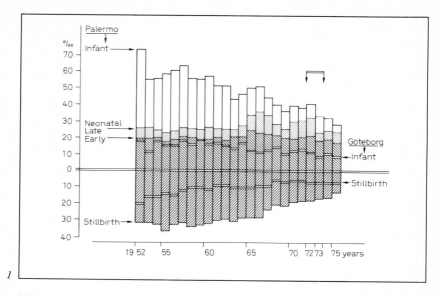

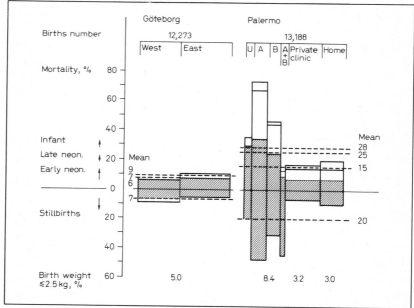

Fig. 1. Perinatal mortality pattern in Göteborg and Palermo during the last decades. Infant mortality also included.

Fig. 2. Stillbirths, early and late neonatal and infant mortality rates in Göteborg and Palermo during period studied. Low birth weight rates included.

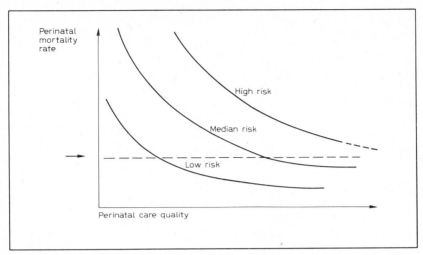

Fig. 3. Schematic relationship between perinatal mortality and perinatal care quality.

care is differentiated in three main parts: one University Hospital and two City Hospitals (together 36%), in 13 private clinics (together 38%), and in home deliveries (25%). Sick newborn infants are referred to either of two children's hospitals.

The overall mortality rates are different according to the various kinds of perinatal care. The four mortality rates: stillbirths rate, early and late neonatal mortality rate, and infant mortality rate for each main place/category are graphically illustrated in figure 2. The proportion of population studied is also indicated for each one.

The Palermo hospitals show relatively high rates, especially Hospital A, the private clinics having the lowest. For the home deliveries, the rates are low, not far from the rates at the two Göteborg hospitals, in spite of being drawn from the lower social groups. The two Göteborg hospitals have the same perinatal mortality rate, though there is a slight difference in the proportions between the two.

Can figures on overall perinatal mortality be used for planning improvement of the perinatal system? Our answer is: not directly. There is naturally an inverse relationship between perinatal mortality and quality of perinatal care, graphically indicated in figure 3, but the character of the perinatal population also exerts a great influence.

Extremely good care of a high-risk population may have the same or even higher mortality rate than mediocre care of a selected low-risk population.

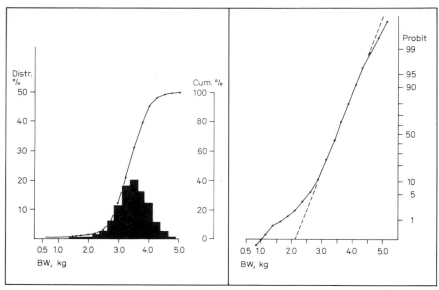

Fig. 4. Birth weight distribution in the Göteborg material given in histogram, cumulative percentage in metric scale and in non-linear 'probit' scale.

Therefore, mortality rate needs to be subdivided into rates for definable perinatal groups after establishing criteria for estimating risks. When considering an overall mortality rate for a given population, geographically defined or perinatal care defined, the distribution of such various risk groups/risk factors within the birth population concerned must be given.

Perinatal Mortality Charts – a Tool for Clinical Evaluation

Based on the analyses in sections III, IV, and V, a combined graphic presentation has been constructed to facilitate the evaluation of existent situations; this is: (a) description of birth population in relation to perinatal risk factors as cumulative percentage distribution, and (b) group-specific mortality rates in relation to perinatal risk factors used.

Basically, a probit scale diagram is used. For the clinician not familiar with the characteristics of a probit scale, the birth weight distribution of the Göteborg material is illustrated in figure 4 as a histogram, a cumulative percentage in metric scale, and in a probit scale.

In the probit scale, deviations in Gaussian distributions or in mixed population are detectable, especially deviations in the lower and upper ends of the distribution. If there is a big 'middle stream', a straight line through 50% will be seen in the condensed middle area. Use of the probit scale for specific mortality rates will also enlarge low rates, making them easily readable, together with high rates of up towards 50%.

Two types of perinatal mortality charts have been constructed: a statistical perinatal chart with total perinatal mortality, and a clinical perinatal mortality chart with stillbirths and neonatal deaths separated.

Statistical perinatal mortality chart. It is well known, and shown in all perinatal surveys, as in the present study, that there is a strong relationship between birth weight and perinatal mortality. Birth weight, being also the most commonly available general measure of the fetus/newborn infant, is thus useful for descriptive population distributions and for group specific mortality rates, when considering the perinatal risk factor.

A birth weight grouping in 250 gram steps with the middle weights 500, 750, 1,000, 1,250, 1,500, 1,750, 2,000, etc., up to 6,000 g and over, has been used in accordance with sections III, IV, and V.

Figure 5a illustrates the utilization of a statistical perinatal chart with birth weight distribution and birth weight specific perinatal rates for three different data bases. The risk is lowest in an area around the mean birth weight, and increases with decreasing birth weight reaching 100% around 700–600 g. At the other end there is a slight to moderate increase for the heavier fetus/newborn infants.

Clinical perinatal mortality chart. In clinical practice, the questions concerning perinatal risks are usually: How high is the risk of remaining *in utero,* i.e. for an intrauterine death? How high is the risk to be born at the specific gestational age, or estimated body size, i.e. for a failure in neonatal adaptation?

Therefore, there is good reason to separate stillbirths and neonatal deaths, although there are some cases when the two overlap. With increased expertise in modern intensive neonatal care in supporting functional adaptation in the early days, deaths related to perinatal conditions often will occur in the late neonatal period. Thus, it seems reasonable to consider and cover the whole neonatal period up to 28 days.

According to the information available and to the desired purpose, birth weight grouping in 250-gram steps, or gestational age grouping in weeks, may be used as a risk factor indicator for descriptive population distributions, and for group-specific rates of stillbirths and of neonatal deaths. Descriptive population distribution is only applied to live births for any general comparable statistic parameter for stillbirths does not exist.

The specific stillbirth rates are calculated from numbers of pregnancies entering the actual risk factor group, as actual 250-gram birth weight groups or gestational week groups, i.e. total births minus small/earlier stillbirths *and* live births. Neonatal mortality rate is calculated from live births of the actual group.

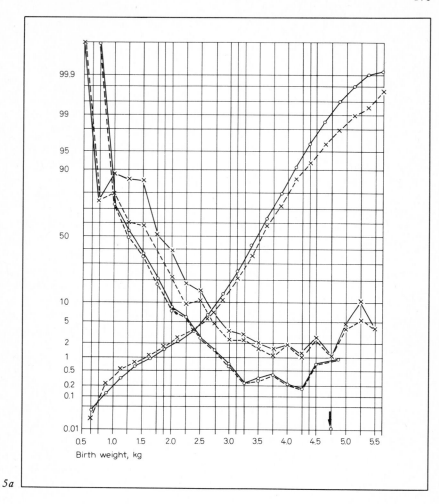

5a

Fig. 5a. Statistical perinatal mortality chart for Göteborg (○) and Palermo (×). Birth weight, grouping in 250 g. Cumulative distribution of singletons' birth weight, total births (low left to top right). Birth weight specific perinatal mortality rates (top left to low right), perinatal mortality (stillbirths, early neonatal deaths), and late perinatal mortality (stillbirths, neonatal deaths up to 28 days). Ordinate: non-linear 'probit' scale. *b* Statistical perinatal mortality chart for Palermo (different places of delivery) and Göteborg (total). Birth weight grouping in 250 g. Cumulative distribution of singletons' birth weights, total births (low left to top right). Birth weight specific late perinatal mortality rates (top left to low right).

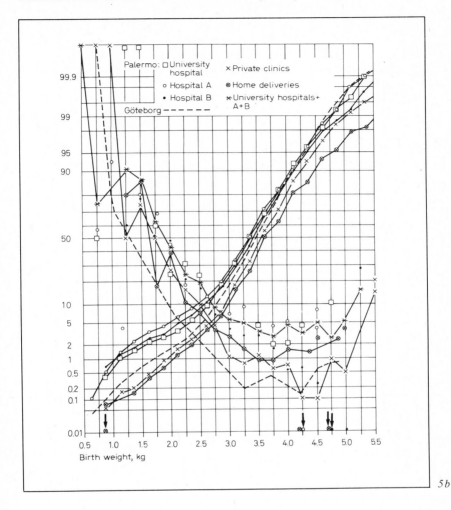

5b

For concentration, and the need for functional context, the group-specific stillbirth rates are placed underneath a live birth distribution – neonatal mortality rates but with negative scale, i.e. increased rates going downwards. Stillbirths not reaching alive the surface of birth may be said to remain below.

Figures 6 and 7 illustrate clinical perinatal mortality charts with birth weight grouping and gestational week grouping, respectively. To be born small/ preterm or to be born heavy/post-term signifies high risk, starting with 100% neonatal mortality from 500 to 700 g or 24–26 weeks (not viable), and certainly ending with 100% intrauterine death not being born.

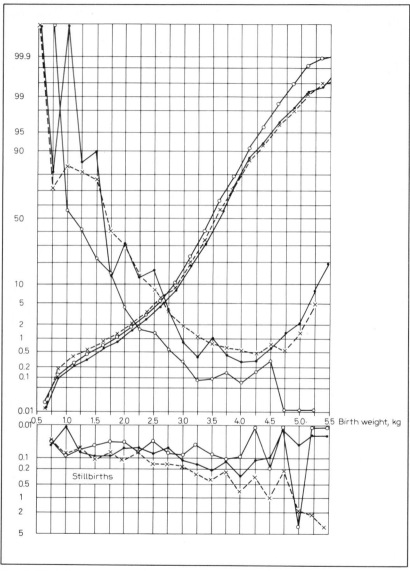

Fig. 6. Clinical perinatal mortality chart for Göteborg total material (○), Palermo total material (×), and Palermo cases with known gestational age (●). Birth weight grouping in 250 g. Cumulative distribution of singleton, live births (low left to top right). Birth weight specific neonatal mortality rates (up to 28 days) calculated on live births (top left to low right). Birth weight specific still birth rates calculated on total number of pregnancies entering actual birth weight group (below with negative scale).

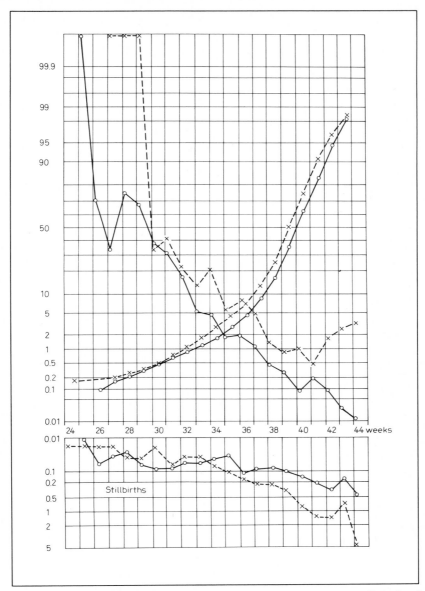

Fig. 7. Clinical perinatal mortality chart for Göteborg (○) and Palermo (×). Gestational age grouping in weeks. Cumulative distribution of singleton, live births (low left to top right). Gestational age specific neonatal mortality rates (up to 28 days), calculated on live births (top left to low right). Gestational age specific stillbirth rates, calculated on total number of pregnancies entering actual week (below with negative scale).

Evaluation in the Statistical Perinatal Mortality Chart

Similar birth weight distribution excludes excess of low birth weight deaths in Palermo. Different birth weight-specific perinatal mortality rates. Due to the heavy incidence of late neonatal deaths in Palermo (see especially section IV), the late perinatal mortality rates (stillbirths and neonatal deaths up to 28 days after birth) are in figure 5a, given together with the ordinary perinatal deaths (stillbirths and neonatal deaths up to 7 days).

The birth weight-specific perinatal mortality rates of the two cities show a pattern in accordance with the above-mentioned general trend. The rates for Palermo are, however, significantly higher in relation to Göteborg, the difference being relatively larger for the area around the median birth weight and is 8–5 times higher. For the lower weights around 1,500 g, the relative differences are less, although the absolute differences are still numerically large. When the late neonatal deaths are included, the differences become bigger especially for the lower birth weights.

The birth weight distribution is similar but some differences are seen: the Palermo material showing a slight shift towards heavier babies — 100 g heavier at the median, a slightly raised lower tail; i.e. there are some more very light babies, but with about the same relative numbers below 2,500 g, and a more pronounced upper tail of heavier babies in the last 10%, pointing to a larger variance for Palermo.

Conclusion. The overall higher perinatal mortality in Palermo cannot be explained by an increased proportion of babies with low birth weight which was our primary hypothesis. The birth weight specific rates are different.

In Palermo, different perinatal care systems have different birth weight distribution/different risk populations, also indicated by higher birth weight specific mortality rates. In figure 5b, the Palermo data are separated for different places of confinement. The birth weight distributions show that the main hospitals are responsible for a definite high-risk perinatal population. There is a big tail of small newborn babies, with 9–6% below 2.5 kg, and the median birth weight is 50 g lower than the Göteborg newborn infant. Both in the private clinics and for home deliveries there are, in general, larger newborn infants and only 3% below 2.5 kg, indicating a low-risk population. For home deliveries, there is a pronounced upper tail, indicating a heavy subpopulation.

Concerning the mortality rates, only the late perinatal mortality rate is given. The hospitals have the highest, especially for median weight groups, which indicates a high-risk population even within this birth weight range. Hospital A has definitely the highest figures. Although the private clinics and the home deliveries have a low-risk population according to the birth weight distribution, the mortality of the median group is higher than in the Göteborg mixed material with few exceptions.

Conclusion. Equal overall mortality rates do not necessarily mean similar situations. Birth weight distribution *and* birth weight specific mortality rate give significantly more information. This principle of analyses also allows us to keep in mind the lower end of the spectrum with the borderline towards abortion and very small immature infants with early neonatal death. Such differentiation will never be equal for places over different time periods, nor between different places/countries.

Evaluation in the Clinical Perinatal Mortality Chart

Stillbirth rates are fairly constant and similar up to 2.5 kg and 33 weeks. Palermo then increases; Göteborg only for gestational age. Neonatal mortality rates are similar for short gestational age then increasing; a difference especially for long gestational age and high birth weight, Palermo having the higher rate. Accelerated intrauterine growth in Palermo.

In figure 6, the values are related to birth weight, and in figure 7 to gestational weeks. The stillbirth rates are fairly constant up to birth weights of 2.5 kg, then Palermo rises but Göteborg slowly drops. When related to gestational age the rate is constant up to 34 weeks, with one stillbirth per 1,000–2,000 pregnancies per week, then a rise in both places and most rapidly in Palermo.

The differences in specific neonatal mortality rates are less pronounced for low gestational age than for low birth weights; but for high gestational age and high birth weights the Göteborg rates drop but the Palermo rates rise, causing a widening difference.

The gestational age chart shows a more 'direct' function of maturity than birth weight (see below), but gestational age is not always obtainable — birth weight being clearly more so. This is the case in the Palermo information. Since gestational age was obtainable only from the standard records in Palermo, figure 7 is for 5,000 deliveries, but figure 6 with birth weight for 12,000 deliveries. In order to show the representativity of the gestational age data, in figure 6 the birth weights of cases with known gestational age are analyzed separately. There is a good agreement in specific neonatal mortality rates, as in birth weight distribution of live births, except for a somewhat reduced number of newborn infants with low birth weight. The stillbirth rates are reduced, especially for the heavier fetuses.

Concerning the distribution of live births, the Palermo subsample of known birth weight and gestational age has a constant higher birth weight and a constant shorter gestational age compared to the Göteborg data, but the slopes of the probit curves are very similar with two pronounced populations especially for gestational age.

Conclusion. Separated stillbirth rate and neonatal mortality rate for 0–28 days, gestational age and birth weight specific, improves the clinical evaluation of perinatal hazards. The differences in the distributions of gestational age and birth weight in the two cities with the pattern of mortality rates indicate an accelerated intrauterine growth of Palermo infants giving a reduced risk at low gestational age and possibly an increased risk for reaching too fast too large a size before delivery.

Functional Causes of Perinatal Deaths

Similar gas exchange disturbances in small newborns, malformations and fetopathies in full-term sized newborn infants. In Palermo, gas exchange disturbances in full-term sized fetus/newborns and a spread of postnatal infections.

In section IV, a simple method of differentiating functional causes of perinatal deaths is presented. The method has primarily two dimensions. One dimension groups main functional causes arranged in usual time sequence of death around the birth for stillbirths and neonatal deaths. The second dimension is a birth weight grouping, the same as in the birth weight distribution and birth weight specific mortality rates.

In the Göteborg sample, gas exchange disturbances below birth weight 1,125 g dominate, while a narrow tail towards the bigger birth weights are mostly associated with malformations or fetopathies. These diagnoses seem to dominate the small-sized stillbirths.

The Palermo picture shows a similar situation for the very small infants as for Göteborg, but there are several gas exchange disturbances as causes of neonatal death in all birth weight groups, and a large number of them among the stillbirths around 3.5-kg birth weight. There is a clear two-population distribution. There are then postnatal infections spread out over all birth weights with some concentration in the middle group 1.5–2.5 kg. Malformations and fetopathies show about the same picture as in Göteborg.

Deviation in intrauterine growth is associated with perinatal risks. In Göteborg, retarded intrauterine growth dominates; in Palermo, accelerated intrauterine growth seems to be of significance.

By the introduction of gestational age, it was obvious that light-for-dates fetuses dominated the Göteborg stillbirths, but this was also found among the neonatal deaths after 33 weeks of gestational age, indicating retarded intrauterine growth.

In Palermo, light-for-dates infants were primarily seen among the neonatal deaths, though the main portion were of appropriate-for-dates infants. The stillbirths are appropriate-for-dates or heavy-for-dates fetuses.

Introduction of the relationship birth weight to birth length (section IV) showed in Göteborg almost a clear cut-off point: a birth weight below the average for actual length, especially among the stillbirths, i.e. signs of intra-uterine hyponutrition, when excluding the smallest fetuses/newborn infants.

Although in Palermo birth length was available only in a reduced number of cases (25%), some tendencies may be pointed out: low weight/length was mostly seen among 2.0–2.5 kg neonatal death infants with postnatal infections, i.e. signs of intrauterine hyponutrition. Disturbed gas exchange in stillbirths and neonatal deaths showed often high weight/length, i.e. sign of intrauterine hyper-nutrition.

Conclusion: It is possible to perform a meaningful grouping in functional causes of perinatal deaths in spite of big differences in the clinical perinatal information obtained. Evaluation of growth and development status in relation to time forms an essential part of such a system.

Birth/Size – Indicator of Intrauterine Growth and Condition of Fetus/Newborn Infant Entering Birth Process/Neonatal Adaptation

Evaluation of growth and development always requires reference to body size and developmental criteria in relation to age. There are principally two kinds of references: population growth pattern and health growth pattern, character-izing the actual population and a useful health standard, respectively, and usu-ally not equal. The growth pattern may be described from the distribution of various factors. Probit analyses are found very useful, directly giving median, percentiles, differentiation of possible subpopulations and, with Gaussian distri-bution, means and standard deviations (SD).

Different population growth patterns. For full-term infants as a group or in age range 37–41 weeks, the distributions are Gaussian. Since there is a high concentration with and around full-term ages, the 'middle stream' distribution of total births gives a fair estimation of the characteristics of the actual birth population, total or subsampled.

The findings in section III are summarized in table I concerning gestational age, birth weight and birth length comparing Palermo to Göteborg, males to females, parity 0 to parity 1, 2; parity > 3 to parity 1, 2; maternal age < 20 and > 35 years to maternal age 20–34 years. By comparing pairs in the mid-part distribution around medians, and lower and upper tails, a visual semi-quantita-tive estimate of the influence of various factors on the preceding intrauterine growth was made. In figure 8, the median values of gestational age and birth weight are plotted.

In the mid-part of the distributions there is, in general, an inverse relation-ship between birth weight and gestational age. For example, the Palermo new-born in relation to the Göteborg newborn, males in relation to females and older

Table I. Visual comparison between pair of distribution of gestational age, birth weight and birth length in 'probit' curves at low tail, mid part and upper tail

Pair	Gestational age						Birth weight						Birth length					
	low		mid		upper		low		mid		upper		low		mid		upper	
	P	G	P	G	P	G	P	G	P	G	P	G	P	G	P	G	P	G
Twin, P/G	=		−				=		−				−		=			
Singletons, P/G	−		−		−		(−)		+		+		=		=		+	
Males/females, P	=		=		(+)		=		+		+		+		(+)		+	
Males/females, G		−		(−)		=		=		+		+		(+)		+		+
Parity																		
0/1, 2 P	(+)		(+)		=		+		−		−		=		−		−	
0/1, 2 G		(−)		(+)		(+)		−		−		−		−		(−)		(−)
≥ 3/1, 2 P	−		=		+		−		+		+		=		=		+	
≥ 3/1, 2 G		−		(−)		(+)		−		=		(+)		−		+		=
Maternal age, years																		
< 20/20−34 P	(−)		=		=		−		−		−		(−)		−		−	
< 20/20−34 G		−		=		−		−		−		−		−		=		−
> 34/20−34 P	−		−		(+)		−		+		+		(−)		(+)		(+)	
> 34/20−34 G		−		−		+		(−)		(+)		+		=		=		(+)

A semiquantitative estimation is used: − (−) = (+) +; negative = lower value, shift to the left; positive = higher value, shift to the right. G = Göteborg; P = Palermo.

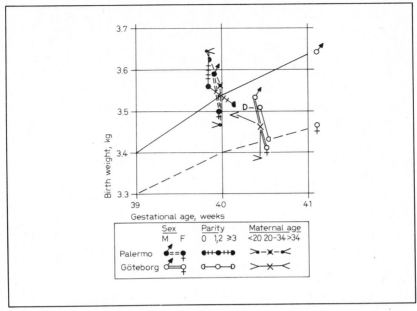

Fig. 8. Median values of distributions of birth weight and of gestational age for males and females, for subsamples with parity 0, 1 + 2, and 3, and for subsamples with maternal age 20, 20–34, and 35 years in the Göteborg and Palermo material. Plotted in an enlarged area the birth weight/gestational age diagram of the Göteborg newborn growth chart.

mothers' infants to mean aged mothers' infants, are bigger and younger. The extreme situation is naturally a pair of twins in relation to singleton.

In the lower tail, there are both a smaller birth weight and a shorter gestational age for all factors related to increased perinatal hazard. This means an increased proportion of the high-risk infants in the selected subsamples. For the upper tail, the situations are about the same as for the mid-parts except for parity > 3 and high maternal age in Palermo, with high birth weight combined with prolonged gestational age. However, paired tails represent only to a certain degree the same individuals.

Conclusion. The similarities clearly dominate the interplay between the various factors within the Göteborg and the Palermo data. A dissimilarity is indicated by a sign, in general, of accelerated intrauterine growth in the Palermo data, and ending in a somewhat earlier delivery.

Similar health growth pattern? Although there are relative differences, the absolute differences in medians are small in relation to the individual variations as illustrated in figure 9 a. The enlarged diagram in figure 8 is fitted into the birth

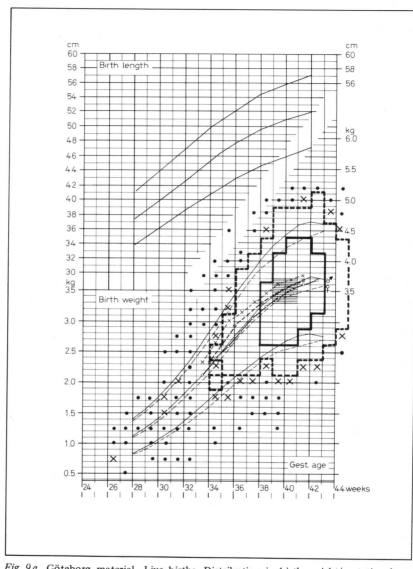

9a

Fig. 9a. Göteborg material. Live births. Distribution in birth weight/gestational age 'cells' 250 g × 1 week superimposed on the birth weight/gestational age diagram of the Göteborg newborn growth chart. Cells with more than 10/1,000 are enclosed within heavy lines, 75.5%; cells with more than 1/1,000 within broken lines, 97.1%; cells with 0.5– 0.9/1,000 marked with ×; cells with 0.1–0.4/1,000 marked with ●. The enlarged area in figure 8 is marked by the grid area. Median birth weight for given gestational week are marked and connected. Uncorrected and corrected median (see text) are used. Palermo:

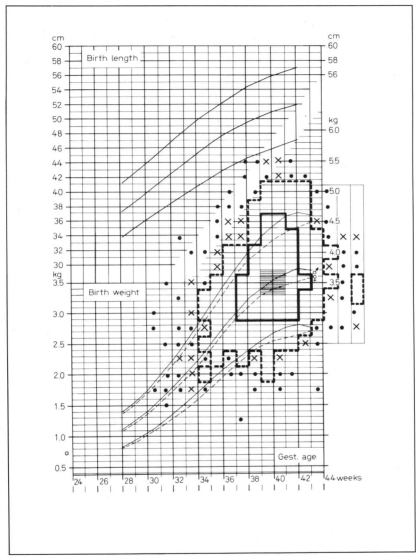

9*b*

uncorrected means (×); corrected means (⊛). Göteborg: uncorrected means (○); corrected means are represented in the mean curves for males and females in the basic diagram. *b* Palermo material, live births. Distribution in birth weight/gestational age 'cells' 250 g × 1 week, superimposed on the birth weight/gestational age diagram of the Göteborg newborn growth chart. Cells with more than 10/1,000 are enclosed within heavy lines, 76.5%; cells with more than 1/1,000 within broken lines, 95.8%; cells with 0.5−9/1,000 marked with ×; cells with 0.1−0.4/1,000 marked ●. The enlarged area in figure 8 is marked by the grid area.

weight/gestational age diagram of the Göteborg newborn growth chart, used in section IV. As a background, the distribution of live births in 'cells' of 250-gram birth weight and 1 week's gestational age are given for the Göteborg data. Cells with more than 10 per 1,000 are marked and cover 75.5% of all births with a birth weight range of 2,625–4,375 g. Cells with more than 1 per 1,000 take 97.1% with a corresponding range of about 2.0–5.0 kg. In figure 10, the Palermo data are presented in the same way. The marked proportions are 76.5 and 95.8%, respectively.

The concentrated distribution of 37–42 weeks, and the possibility of wrongly estimating the gestational age by ± one interval, distort the true distributions, although in a limited number of cases. Especially for 33–35 weeks of gestation, there is a large upper tail distribution in practically all birth data, as there is in the present data in spite of careful scrutiny of the raw data (section III). By exclusion from the total sample, the visually estimated subsample portions, the large upper tails as well as the smaller lower tails, the median value may be corrected to correspond to the estimated true sample. This technique has been used in constructing the standard newborn growth chart of the Göteborg, data, used in section IV. The newborn growth pattern may also be considered as reflecting intrauterine growth, although it is made up by appropriate newborn infants born before term for some reason. The same technique has been used in the Palermo material. The uncorrected and corrected median growth curves are drawn for both the Göteborg and Palermo material in figure 9 a.

The *Palermo* data also show, after correction, an accelerated growth pattern, the time differences being successfully somewhat bigger, ending up as around 1 week difference. Due to the shape of the curves, the differences, however, in birth weight for a given gestational week decrease. The median Palermo baby is 100 g heavier than the Göteborg baby, but is born 5 days earlier. This relationship decreases the influence of different growth rates on the actual birth weight.

Adding the fact that Palermo women are shorter than Göteborg women, with an estimated mean difference of 5–10 cm, the results are even more intriguing and lead to the following speculative considerations:

Accelerated intrauterine growth, especially in short mothers with a small final intrauterine space, stimulates an earlier delivery, overriding usual initiation mechanisms. However, before delivery is initiated, there is a risk of disproportionate development between fetus and birth canal, causing an increased risk for stillbirths and neonatal deaths due to disturbed gas exchange. Especially is this so in fetus/newborn infants with high birth weight as seen in the Palermo data (section IV).

If an early preterm delivery is mainly caused by an incompetent cervix, the tendency for the small preterm babies in Palermo to have a shorter gestational age, but about the same birth weight compared to Göteborg, may also be explained by an early accelerated intrauterine growth (section IV).

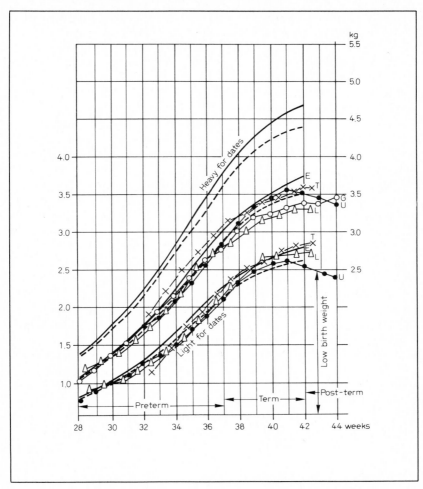

Fig. 10. Some commonly used birth weight/gestational age standards with recommended borderlines to light-for-date. E = *Engström and Falconer* (6), −2 SD (2½ percentile) boys (————) and girls (-----); G (boys and girls) = *Gruenwald* (5), only mean value curve; L (boys) = *Lubchenco et al.* (2), 10th percentile; T (boys) = *Thomson et al.* (3), 5th percentile; U (boys and girls) = *Usher and McLean* (4), −2 SD (2½ percentile).

These tentatively suggested biological mechanisms indicate that the new-born growth pattern found in the Palermo material cannot be considered as an optimal growth pattern. The health growth pattern must be closer to the Göteborg pattern, perhaps even with somewhat lower birth weight/gestational age due to the shorter mothers of Palermo. Further study is needed. In the meantime, we have considered it appropriate to use the Göteborg reference for the clinical evaluation of individual newborn infants in Palermo. Possible reference differences will have a limited significance due to the big individual variations. On the other hand, the basic mechanism of accelerated growth has wide general implications (see below).

In the *Göteborg* data, the main risk factor seems to be the opposite – a retarded intrauterine growth, with light-for-date and light-for-length infants. Even here a standard is required. In the literature, several different reference criteria of light-for-date infants have been recommended: *Lubchenco et al.* (2), 10th percentile; *Thomson et al.* (3), 5th percentile; *Usher and McLean* (4), −2 SD; *Engström and Falconer* (6), also −2 SD = $2^{1}/_{2}$ percentile. When plotted in a birth weight/gestational age diagram, as in figure 10, it is obvious, however, that the differences between the actual values are small, if there are any, due to different mean/median values in the reference material. This signifies that in the different studies the same kind of clinical entity of retarded intrauterine growth has been differentiated independently of the mean/median values.

On the other hand, since there is a rapid drop in the distribution around this level, the precise location will have a great numerical influence on differentiated cases, although the clinical significance will be small. As usual in biological data, there is no clear-cut point, or level, between normality and pathology. For clinical evaluation it is more useful to have some kind of continuous scale which can be given risk loads. We have found SD scores from the mean birth weight for actual gestational age of a health growth pattern very useful (7). Since the SDs seem to be related to the order of the means percentage, or fraction of the corresponding age mean, they are also meaningful in both directions – for retarded as well as for accelerated growth.

Conclusion. The birth size/age has a significant impact on risk evaluation not only for the very small and preterm babies, but also along the newborn growth pattern in the whole range. Birth weight has an important impact other than as an indicator of maturity, for it reflects also velocity and quality of intrauterine growth and thus is a useful indicator of the perinatal risk factor.

Analysis of the relationship between different factors – such as birth weight to gestational age, and to birth length – lead, however, to increase accuracy in differentiation. Since there is clinically no clear cut-off point between normality and pathology, continuous scales are suggested with SD scores or percentages of mean values.

The upper part of the often-seen two population distribution in birth weight per gestational week, in the range of 32−35 weeks, we suggest be excluded, as it is considered to be the effect of miscalculation of gestational age as well as the smaller, lower part. A possible group of newborn infants with accelerated intrauterine growth may also form a portion of this upper part. If so, it should also be excluded from the health growth pattern in order to be able to detect these newborn infants in clinical practice. The relationship between birth weight and birth length has been found very useful, and here the possible uncertainty of gestational age is excluded. Application of mathematical models will still further improve our knowledge of biological events, and our evaluation of individual cases in clinical practice. (The suggested method of graphical corrections will be further described in an analysis of a Swedish newborn material; in preparation, to be published elsewhere).

Intrauterine Growth Is One of the Key Issues in Perinatal Hazards

An *interrupted* intrauterine growth (i.e. a *preterm* delivery) implies obviously an increased risk, especially for a failure in neonatal adaptation due to a low degree of maturity achieved. The risk increases with shorter gestational age, and is 100% at 24–28 weeks. Preterm deliveries are present in both Göteborg and Palermo, and form numerically in Göteborg the main portion of perinatal casualties.

A *prolonged* intrauterine growth (i.e. a *post-term* delivery) means also an increased risk with time (theoretically towards 100%), and is always a reality. In Göteborg, preventive measures during antenatal care seem to have reached a fairly effective stage.

Slow or *retarded* intrauterine growth has attracted an increasing interest and significance in the perinatal field during the last decade. It is also the dominating factor, besides preterm deliveries, in Göteborg. Studies in our laboratories have shown metabolic disturbances in these newborn infants (7).

Fast or *accelerated* intrauterine growth contributes in part to the clinical entity of diabetic fetopathy. The present studies indicate that accelerated intrauterine growth is a basal risk factor in Palermo.

Deviations in intrauterine growth, in both a negative and a positive direction, have been found in the present study to have such an impact on perinatal hazards that intrauterine growth must be considered a key issue in the perinatal field. Retardation as well as acceleration have to be further studied for cause and the course aiming at early diagnosis, means of possible correction, indication for intervention and, ultimately, for prevention. Since several factors significantly related to perinatal mortality/morbidity are associated with disturbed intrauterine growth, studies of underlying mechanisms must lead to improvement in outcome.

The influence of maternal body size, maternal age and parity need certainly to be further studied, and nutritional factors are of great importance. Hypernutrition, especially of carbohydrates in the pregnant Palermo women, tentatively is thought to be a contributory factor to the high perinatal hazards. Inadequate nutrition and/or anxiety and distress in unfavorable micro-environments are possible causes of retarded intrauterine growth. Drugs, alcohol, smoking are other significant factors.

The low perinatal hazard for high-standard socioeconomic family groups and high hazard for low-standard socioeconomic groups are certainly multifactorially influenced, and need to be analyzed in order to find the key causal factors. The even birth weight distribution, with only a small lower tail and very little upper tail, in subsamples of socioeconomic standards, indicates undisturbed intrauterine growth in most cases, with a balance between accelerating and retarding factors. The subsample of low socioeconomic standards shows an uneven distribution. Significant relationship between social grouping and perinatal hazard *per se* does not lead to improvement in perinatal care, but gives pointers towards factors in need of study and attack.

Conclusion. The findings in these studies point to the importance of intrauterine growth, not only the cut-off time (i.e. the degree of maturity reached at birth), but also the quality of growth and development. Effort to improve perinatal care (i.e. reduced perinatal hazard) must include this issue. Possible relationships with underlying mechanisms to the sex of infant, low and high maternal age, parity 0 and high parity, low socioeconomic grouping have to be further studied and analyzed.

General Conclusions

Comparison of Göteborg-Palermo

The perinatal mortality is different, and three to four times higher in Palermo than in Göteborg. Such a difference was expected, and formed a basis for the study. The perinatal care system in Palermo covers the full spectrum, whereas Göteborg is at the other extreme: two maternity hospitals with 2,500–3,000 deliveries per year, which aim to cover all demands for a population of half a million.

The functional causes of death in the two cities have small preterm newborns, malformations and fetopathies in common. Palermo has differently a large proportion of gas exchange disturbances, especially in full-term infants, and postnatal infections, especially in infants with birth weights of 1.5–2.5 kg. In Göteborg, the signs of retarded intrauterine growth are common in perinatal deaths, and in Palermo, there are indications of accelerated intrauterine growth as a further basal factor.

The big differences in mortality rates, and functional causes of death between the different places of deliveries in Palermo are certainly, to a great extent, due to selection in the actual birth populations. The effect of possible differences due to matching perinatal care quality to the demand cannot be evaluated from the present data.

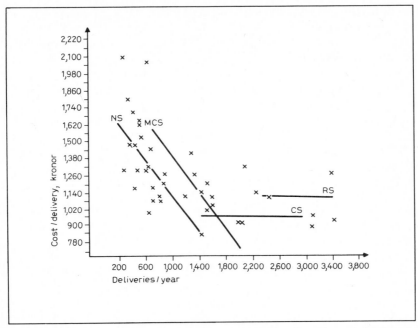

Fig. 11. Swedish perinatal care investigation (1973): Cost/benefit analysis. Average cost per delivery in relation to hospital size in number of deliveries per year. Regression lines are calculated for general hospitals (NS), small central general hospitals (MCS), central general hospitals (CS), and regional hospitals (RS). Average hospital delivery cost in Sweden = 99.98 kr. (1972). Förlossningsvardens organisation: Sverige, Socialstyrelsen 35, Stockholm 1973.

In Göteborg, too, differences, although much smaller, are found between the two hospitals. Primarily, the two institutions were considered to be equal both in birth population, and in care. The proportions, however, between stillbirths and neonatal deaths differ. After scrutiny of individual cases, and in applying the WHO criteria of live birth, there seems no significant explanation for the difference. The findings indicate slight differences in risk populations within the total birth populations. There are some differences in the differentiation of mild symptoms, and though there may be slight differences in care, this cannot be evaluated from the available data.

The differences between Göteborg and Palermo in perinatal mortality can, to some extent, be explained by the increased proportion of both low and high maternal ages and of high parities in Palermo, each separated in groups having a high mortality rate. The higher proportion of parity 0 in Göteborg must be considered as influencing a comparable lower risk factor.

It is reasonable to assume that the evolved perinatal care system in Göteborg is of definite significance. It might be of interest to point out that a recent cost/benefit investigation in Sweden has shown that normal deliveries in small hospitals result in a much higher cost than in a medium-sized hospital; and higher still than in regional maternity hospitals where there are concentrations of risk populations together with the ordinary birth population (fig. 11). The perinatal mortality rates in the regional and large hospitals with 2,000–3,000 deliveries per year are also lower than the mean for the whole country (*Karlberg*, 1976). The general policy is to aim towards maternity hospitals of this size, or at least over 1,700 deliveries per year, both for maintaining a sufficient high quality of care, and for the economical reasons that are apparent.

The comparative high standard of living in Sweden must also have an influence. On the other hand, the findings of the present study indicate that the birth population in Palermo puts special demands on the perinatal care system due to possible accelerated intrauterine growth generally present. The higher frequency of Cesarean section in Palermo compared to Göteborg has been noted, but there is also a high incidence of postnatal infections in newborn infants with birth weights of 1.5–2.5 kg in the private clinics. Is there, perhaps, an increased risk for light-for-dates infants in the higher socioeconomic groups?

The study shows the importance of 'communicating chambers', for example: (1) the distribution of risk births; (2) balancing negative and positive factors with a resultant optimum in the middle, for instance, in intrauterine growth, and (3) for the need for further studies to increase our knowledge of basic underlying mechanisms.

The use of perinatal mortality figures for estimation of priorities in improvement of perinatal care. Let us go back to the question in the beginning of this section; study of the key factors in perinatal mortality should lead to good planning for the improvement of perinatal care. Crude perinatal mortality rates have limited value. With risk factor/system grouping of the birth population and of the mortality rates, and with a simple grouping of functional causes of death, a reasonable estimation of priorities for the improvement of perinatal care can be made. The diagram similar to the one in figure 3 may be used as a base for illustration (fig. 12).

In Göteborg: the improvement of care of the very small newborn babies to the level that available resources allow. The monitoring prenatal functional disturbances. The diagnosis of retarded intrauterine growth and then emphasizing the necessity to select an optimal time and mode of delivery. Can the number of malformations be reduced? should be asked.

In Palermo: the improvement of the perinatal care of the full-term infant with especial emphasis on feto-maternal factors, and on the possible need of resuscitation of any newborn baby. The combatance of perinatal and postnatal infections. These priorities hold for all the places of confinement. The differ-

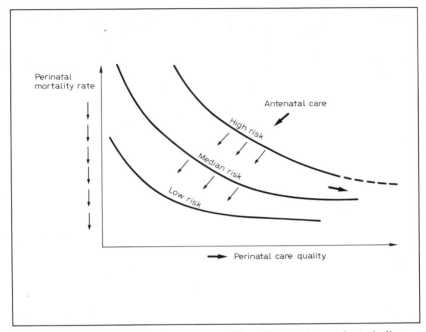

Fig. 12. Suggested priorities in improvement efforts illustrated in a schematic diagram of the relationship between perinatal mortality rate and perinatal care quality.

ences in perinatal mortality between these in Palermo depend obviously to a great deal on the selected birth populations. The significance of possible variations in the quality of perinatal care cannot be evaluated from the present data.

For both Göteborg and Palermo, antenatal care aiming to reduce high-risk birth populations is a key issue. The study results indicate that special attention should be paid to different sides of 'the valley of the shadow of birth' — in Göteborg to the intrauterine growth retardation side; in Palermo to the intrauterine growth acceleration side.

In both cities, too, much emphasis needs to be made on the avoidance of the newborn infant getting too early or too late into 'the valley'. This stresses the importance of knowing the time of the start of *each* pregnancy. This information is a basic key in the aim to give each fetus and newborn baby optimal support, and to guard them through the perinatal period to an intact survival.

In figure 13, the main risk areas are indicated using the birth weight, birth weight/gestational age diagram of the newborn growth chart: too early delivery and too late delivery, retarded intrauterine growth, and accelerated intrauterine growth — the last area being less defined at present.

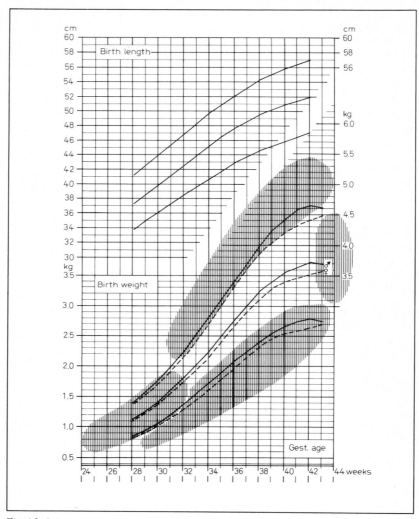

Fig. 13. Schematic indication of the main risk area in perinatal hazards. Base: the birth weight/gestational age diagram of the newborn growth chart.

Summary

The findings presented in the preceding sections have been evaluated from the clinical point of view. The big differences recorded in perinatal mortality rates between Göteborg and Palermo, and between the different categories of perinatal care in Palermo, need, for clinical evaluation, the combination of a distribution of risk factors within the actual birth population, and the risk factor specific mortality rates. Perinatal mortality charts for facilitating such analyses have been designed. As the primary risk factor, birth weight grouping in 250-gram ranges with mid-points of 0.75, 1.00, 1.25, 1.50, 2.00, 2.25, 2.50, 2.75, etc. have been used in accordance with preceding sections. The influence of a somewhat pronounced tendency to read off even figures is excluded, and the group range of 250 g gives a clinically useful differentiation.

The higher perinatal mortality rates recorded in Palermo cannot be explained by an increased incidence of low birth weights, for, on the contrary, the newborn infants are in general somewhat heavier in Palermo than in Göteborg. The birth weight-specific perinatal mortality rates are all higher in Palermo.

Low-risk populations, but with still high specific mortality rates, may give low overall perinatal mortality rates as in private clinics and home deliveries in Palermo.

A separation of specific stillbirth rates and neonatal mortality rates (up to 28 days), as in the clinical perinatal mortality chart presented, improves the clinical evaluation of perinatal hazards. It is suggested that stillbirth rates be calculated from numbers of pregnancies entering the actual risk factor group, as actual 250-gram birth weight groups or gestational week groups, i.e. total births minus smaller/earlier stillbirths *and* live births. Neonatal mortality rate is calculated from live births of the actual group.

Such findings can later be used as a reference in clinical practice for assessing the risk for a continued pregnancy, intrauterine existence, for interrupted pregnancy, failure in neonatal adaptation, and for evolving priorities. Gestational age grouping is a more direct and 'cleaner' risk factor related to degrees of maturity status than birth weight grouping, which also includes deviations of intrauterine growth.

The main functional causes of perinatal deaths grouping and in birth weight gives a useful two-dimensional differentiation. When combined with evaluation of birth size/age, i.e. birth weight to gestational age and birth weight to birth length, further information was obtained which showed the importance of assessing previous intrauterine growth in relation to velocity and quality, for a better understanding of perinatal events. The necessary reference for the evaluation of growth is discussed in terms of population growth pattern and health growth pattern.

The similarities and dissimilarities in perinatal hazards between the two cities studies may be summarized as follows:

(1) Early interrupted pregnancies – shortened intrauterine existence – i.e. small preterm newborn infants, are common to both.

(2) Malformations (embryopathies) and fetopathies are also common to both, especially in full-term neonatal deaths and early stillbirths. These dominate the situation in Göteborg due to the very low number of other perinatal deaths within these graphs.

(3) In Palermo, on the other hand, disturbed gas exchange and postnatal infections dominate the picture.

(4) Analyses of intrauterine growth, excluding the small preterm newborn infants, show in Göteborg over-representation of retarded intrauterine growth and in Palermo, an indication of accelerated intrauterine growth with increased complications in delivery and more demands on the perinatal care system.

(5) In Palermo, retarded intrauterine growth seems to be related to a susceptibility to infection.

(6) The hazard of post-term delivery seems to be reduced more actively in Göteborg than in Palermo.

(7) In Palermo, there are higher incidences of high parities and high maternal age which explains in some measure the differences in outcome. Differences in perinatal care, and also in standard of living, are considered to be of significant importance.

The influences of maternal age, parity, socioeconomic grouping, and possibly also sex, are suggested to operate basically over mechanisms related to intrauterine growth, the length of intrauterine existence, and the velocity and the quality of growth. The need for further studies of underlying mechanism is emphasized. Mathematical models including intrauterine growth factors and risk factors will be one important tool. There is a need for increased accuracy in the determination of risk areas.

Already priorities for the improvement of perinatal care aimed to reduce perinatal hazards can be set from the results of the study.

References

1   *Smith, C.A.:* The valley of the shadow of birth. Am. J. Dis. Child. *82:* 171 (1951).

2   *Lubchenco, L.O.; Hausman, C.; Dressler, M., and Boyd, E.:* Intrauterine growth as estimated from liveborn birth-weight data at 24 to 42 weeks of gestation. Pediatrics *32:* 793 (1963).

3   *Thomson, A.M.; Billewics, W.Z., and Hytten, F.E.:* The assessment of fetal growth. J. Obstet. Gynaec. Br. Commonw. *75:* 903 (1968).

4   *Usher, R. and McLean, F.:* Intrauterine growth of live-born caucasian infants at sea level: standards obtained from measurements in 7 dimensions of infants born between 25 and 44 weeks of gestation. J. Pediat. *74:* 901 (1969).

5   *Gruenwald, P.:* Growth of the human fetus. I. Normal growth and its variation. Am. J. Obstet. Gynec. *94:* 1112 (1966).

6   *Engström, L. and Falconer, B.:* En jämförelse mellan svenska nyfödda barns längd och vikt 1911–1920 och 1956–1957. Sv. Läkartidn *57:* 1759 (1960).

7   *Gustafson, A.; Kjellmer, I.; Olegård, R., and Victorin, L.:* Nutrition in low birth weight infants. I. Intravenous injection of fat emulsion. Acta paediat. scand. *61:* 149 (1972).

Prof. *P. Karlberg,* Department of Pediatrics, University of Göteborg, East Hospital, *S–416 85 Göteborg* (Sweden)

Prof. *A. Priolisi,* Child Health Institute, University of Palermo, Via Lancia DiGrolo 10 B *Palermo* (Italy)

Section VII

Monogr. Paediat., vol. 9, pp. 193–197 (Karger, Basel 1977)

Conclusions

F. Falkner

It has appeared that there are two main areas concerned in such a study as this: epidemiological and biomedical-clinical, with ancillary care and resources. Though there is no, nor should there be any, clear division between them.

Epidemiologically, we have experience of the two approaches (basically) to data collection — a specially mounted research project (Palermo), or the use of a clinical record generated on a routine basis (Göteborg). Each has advantages and disadvantages.

In terms of the reporting of mortality, there are apparent differences in the conventions applied in classifying stillbirths and deaths following live birth, and this emphasizes the advantage of using perinatal mortality (as opposed to infant mortality) as a measure of outcome. The measurements of maturity (and particularly birth weight) were subject to an element of digit preference, and because of the shape of the birth weight distribution curve, the use of the 2,500-gram borderline between 'low' and 'higher' weight births tends to bias estimates of the crude form of the birth weight distribution.

When the various measures of maturity are compared, birth weight is by far the most useful as a predictor of mortality, with gestational age providing some further information. Birth length and head circumference contribute very little extra, however.

Maturity is the most sensitive indicator of mortality. Our data about maternal age, parity, social class, complications of pregnancy and delivery, and so on, are in agreement with most of the existing literature. The general form of the maturity/mortality relationship is similar in both cities and, in particular, the linear decline of mortality (expressed on a probit scale) with maturity in low maturity births is a common feature. This suggests a useful analogy with dosage response analysis in biological assay, maturity being a kind of generalized stimulus or dosage. Our results also establish that a naturally occurring population consists of a mixture of two main distributions in terms of maturity.

The effect of missing data on the form of the relationships which we have studied is worth emphasizing. Given that, say, 95% of the population is covered (a high figure for epidemiological studies), and the missing 5% is concentrated on the deaths, the relationship between mortality and other factors (e.g. head circumference) is seriously distorted. This point seems to have gone virtually unnoticed in the epidemiological literature.

At Palermo, there were large differences in mortality between the various places of confinement, and clearly a part of these differences was due to population selection effects (e.g. higher social classes use private clinics more often than lower social classes). In a system in which there is more than one type of place of confinement, the results from a single place of confinement (e.g. hospital) need not necessarily apply to the whole population.

Regarding maturity indicators in the two cities, birth weight, gestational age, and birth length were compared as were the joint distributions of birth weight and gestational age and birth weight and birth length. Median birth weights are similar in the two cities, but Göteborg shows less variation. The proportion of low birth weight infants interestingly appears to be nearly identical. In the highest weights, there is a much higher percentage of very heavy infants in Palermo, and this causes the greater variability there – a quite atypical pattern when compared to distibutions in the UK and USA or, indeed, Sweden.

Low birth weight and short length infants appear very similar in the two cities as regards their proportion of all births. Though the Palermo infants have a shorter gestational period of some 4–5 days – a finding consistent with other studies of race – when compared to Göteborg, the cumulative gestational age plots have the same shape as for birth weight and length which is consistent.

Infants with short gestational periods weigh more in Palermo. And again, on average, short Palermo infants weigh more; however, long infants weigh more in Göteborg.

It seems as if more growth occurred in each gestational week among the Palermo fetuses – that the week was more 'biologically intense'. It would seem worthwhile to study in depth this possible biological attribute, or complex heterogeneous genetic background, of the Palermo population that could contribute, too, to the unusual shape of the cumulative distribution curves of birth weights.

We aimed to derive some conclusion that would point the way to lowering the perinatal mortality rate and suggesting priorities for using available resources or obtaining them – the biomedical-clinical-care-resources area.

We have found large differences in mortality. These are greatest in relative terms for the higher birth weight groups. In terms of cause of death, much of the disadvantage at Palermo is associated with deaths due to infection in these higher birth weight classes.

On the other hand, when one is presented, as at Göteborg, with a small number of virtually solely immature, low birth weight infants, or those with

Table I. Distribution of births in terms of multiplicity, birth weight, and outcome of delivery. Rate per 1,000 live and still births

Outcome	Multiplicity			
	1		2 or more	
	BW below 2,501 g	BW above 2,500 g	BW below 2,501 g	BW above 2,500 g
a) All records				
Late fetal death	5.2	13.2	0.3	0.3
Early neonatal death	6.4	5.1	1.7	0.2
Late neonatal death	4.7	4.7	1.9	0.1
Survived 1 month	28.3	911.6	7.0	8.8
b) Standard Records				
Late fetal death	4.0	12.7	0.5	0.5
Early neonatal death	10.1	7.1	2.8	0.3
Late neonatal death	7.6	6.2	3.5	0.2
Survived 1 month	26.0	898.1	6.6	13.4
c) Edited Standard Records				
Late fetal death	5.0	12.1	0.2	0.2
Early neonatal death	7.1	5.8	1.9	0.4
Late neonatal death	5.0	5.0	1.7	0.2
Survived 1 month	28.5	911.8	8.1	7.1

embryopathy or fetopathy, reward for the specific important resources and effort available at that period in time is comparatively small. Limited resources, then, need to be concentrated where they are most effective, and they are probably not, initially, in this context.

The relatively favorable record for deliveries in private clinics and at home at Palermo is both unexpected and important. Bearing in mind the absence of many basic facilities in the former, the low mortality in private clinics suggests there is a strong 'social class' affect associated perhaps with better nutritional and environmental conditions during pregnancy. The low mortality for home deliveries cannot be attributed to favorable social and economic conditions (the reverse is probably true). Perhaps the home confinements run less risk of infection. However, for these two places of delivery, the record at Palermo is comparable to that at Göteborg, notwithstanding the relatively undeveloped nature of the maternity and pediatric services which are available.

The nature of the antenatal care is reflected to some extent by the distribution of cases in terms of complications of pregnancy and by the mortality associated with each such grade. In general, the greater the quantity and/or the better the quality of antenatal care, the greater the extent and the lower the average level of severity.

The gap between the Palermo and Göteborg populations increases as the birth weight and gestational age increase with regard to perinatal mortality/birth weight and perinatal mortality/gestational age. This indicates that available and potential resources at Palermo need to be applied to the whole birth weight/ gestational age range. This is especially so at a particular part of the range where the mortality relative to Göteborg is notably high. Late neonatal and infant death rates are high, too, in Palermo, indicating the need for action in the neonatal period and on to one year.

Two major groups of perinatal causes of death occur in Palermo — gas-exchange disturbances and infection. Both, to some extent, require intervention by far more than medical expertise. Gas-exchange problems are based on a complex multifactorial base, the interaction of some mechanisms involved not being known. One example of the complexity is that good antenatal and post-natal care to some degree can prevent or reduce the incidence of these distur-bances. Thus, it seems that we are talking about a whole perinatal care system.

The infection problem at Palermo goes one step further in the clear need to educate and involve the whole community, and that community's whole 'child health care' approach.

From the more clinical point of view, perinatal mortality charts were des-igned to help the analysis of what lay behind the big differences in perinatal mortality rates between Göteborg and Palermo, clinical evaluation and the distri-bution of risk factors. The higher perinatal mortality rates in Palermo cannot be explained on the increased incidence of low birth weights, and the birth weight-specific perinatal mortality rates are all higher in Palermo. Low-risk populations that still have high specific mortality rates may show low overall perinatal mor-tality rates as in Palermo's private clinics and home deliveries.

The clinical evaluation of perinatal hazards is improved by use of the clinical perinatal mortality chart presented by separating specific stillbirth and neonatal mortality rates. These findings can be used in clinical settings in order to assess various risks. For example, for a continued pregnancy, a failure in neonatal adaptation, and so forth.

The main causes of perinatal death when combined with the evaluation of birth size showed the importance of assessing previous intrauterine growth in relation to velocity and quality and for a better impression of perinatal events.

There were similarities and dissimilarities in perinatal hazard in the two cities. Small preterm newborn infants, embryopathies, and fetopathies are com-mon to both — especially for the latter two in full-term neonatal death and early stillbirth. Clearly, these dominate in Göteborg where there are low numbers of other perinatal deaths in these groups. In Palermo, retarded intrauterine growth seems to be related to susceptibility to infection, and the post-term delivery hazards are less in Göteborg than Palermo. Here, there are higher incidences of high parities and high maternal age which, in part, may explain this. Clearly, perinatal care and standard of living differences have notable impact.

Maternal age, parity, and socioeconomic factors seem to operate over the basic mechanisms involved in intrauterine growth, its length, its speed, and its quality. Thus, there is a pressing need to study these underlying mechanisms. Mathematical models based on risk and intrauterine growth factors will surely be useful tools. Already the study has shown priority areas for the improvement of perinatal care with the aim of reducing the incidence of perinatal hazards.

Finally, it is to be hoped that the results of the study will provide pointers for priorities in the improvement of perinatal care in different situations, and show the benefit of assessing the relationships of the key factors involved in perinatal mortality.

A much-respected obstetrician once remarked, in praising the advances of neonatology, that it should now be the aim in obstetrics to be less reliant on the skills of the neonatologist in saving the newborn infant in serious trouble and deliver intact high-quality infants. And outcome is what we should focus on. The worst is death, pre-, peri-, or postnatally. And epidemiologically speaking, if one escapes death and does not become a statistic — contributing to the stillbirth rate, perinatal or infant mortality, then one is a survivor. But how intact a survivor?

This leads to what the team involved in this study feel should be a next and further step: to follow up — initially to the first 5 years of life — the outcome of these survivors. Hopefully, a large proportion will be healthy. But what proportion will not be, and what will the relationship of various non-intact or pathological factors and features be to the various key factors and patterns uncovered in this study? Hopefully, some of these questions can be answered by moving into a further phase of our investigations.

Prof. *F. Falkner*, MD, FRCP, Director, Fels Research Institute, *Yellow Springs, OH 45387* (USA)

Appendices

Appendix 1

Summary of Information Collected in the Göteborg and Palermo Surveys

Available data	Göteborg	Palermo prospective survey	retrospective survey		
1. Mother					
Name and address	+	+	U	P	R
Case record No.	+	+	U	P	R
Date of birth	+	+	U	P	R
District of normal residence	(+)	+	U	P	R
2. Mother's obstetric history for each previous pregnancy					
Date of delivery		+			
Place of delivery		+			
Multiplicity		+			
Birth weight		+			
Number of miscarriages	+	+	U	P	
Number of stillborn	+	+	U	P	
Number of liveborn	+	+	U	P	
Number of liveborn dying within 7 days	+	+	U	P	
Number of liveborn dying within 28 days		+	U	P	
Number of liveborn dying within 1 year		+	U	P	
3. Present pregnancy					
1st day of LMP	+	+	U	P	
Duration of pregnancy	+	+	U	P	
a) Certain					
b) Uncertain	+				
c) Characteristics of menstrual					
period and cycle		+	U	P	
Antenatal care					
Detailed monthly analysis		+			
Gestational age at 1st visit	+	+			
Number of visits where/who	+	+			
4. Complication of pregnancy					
(including relevant maternal diseases)	+	+	U	P	
5. Delivery					
Place of delivery	+	+	U	P	(R)
Assistance at birth	(+)	+	U	P	
Multiplicity of birth	+	+	U	P	R
Mode of presentation	+	(+)	(U)	(P)	
Method of delivery	+	+	U	P	
Complications of delivery	+	+	U	P	
Obstetric procedures	+	+	U	P	

Available data	Göteborg	Palermo prospective survey	retrospective survey		
6. *Infant*					
Date of birth	+	+	U	P	R
Sex	+	+	U	P	R
Birth weight	+	+	U	P	R
Birth length	+	+	U		
Head circumference	+				
Umbilical cord anomalies	+	+	U	P	
a) Stillbirths	+	+	U	P ·	R
Maceration/cause of death	+	+	(U)	(P)	(R)
b) Liveborn	+	+	U	P	R
1. Condition at birth	+	M:+	(U)	(P)	
Apgar score at 5 min	+				
Resuscitation procedure	+	M:+	(U)	(P)	
Morbidity	+	(+)	(U)	(P)	
Neonatal procedures	+	(+)	(U)	(P)	
2. Mortality 0–7 days	+	+	U	P	R
Mortality 7–28 days	+	+	U	P	R
Cause of death	+	+	U	P	R
7. *Socioeconomic and family background*					
Mother					
Height	(+)	(+)			
Weight – before delivery		(+)			
Weight – after delivery		(+)			
Date of marriage		+	U		R
Marital status	+	+	U	P	R
Age of finishing full-time education		+	(U)	(P)	(R)
Employment before pregnancy			U	P	R
Employment before/during pregnancy	M:+	+			
Smoking habits		+			
Father					
Height		(+)			
Weight		(+)			
Age of finishing full-time education		+			
Occupation	M:+	+	U	P	R
Income (from tax declaration)	(+)				
Parents' country of birth	+				

+ In all cases; (+) in some cases or restricted information; M:+ only in case of death. For Palermo retrospective survey: U = University Hospital; P = Public Hospitals (A and B); R = births registration.

Appendix 2

The Application of a Randomized Editing Procedure to the Standard Records at Palermo

Four distinct types of records — Standard, University Hospital, Public Hospital, and Statistics Office — were employed in the Palermo survey. The information available varies between the different types of record, with by far the greatest number of items being included on the Standard Records. Thus, for many aspects of the survey, the only source of information are the Standard Records, which cover only some 43.8% of the births. The question then arises as to whether conclusions derived from an analysis of the Standard Records can be applied with confidence to the complete population.

On general grounds, it can be asserted that the type of record available for any particular birth was *not* determined by a process which can be regarded in any sense as random. The subjective view of the survey workers is that the more 'difficult' type of birth was more likely to have been covered with the Standard Records. Multiplicity, outcome of delivery, and birth weight are three items of information which are included on each type of record. The distributions of these three items, excluding a small proportion of missing observations, in the whole population and in the Standard Records are given below in table Ia and b, respectively. There are very highly significant differences in the distribution of all three factors, which confirm that the Standard Records are biased in favor of low weight, multiple births and of stillbirths and neonatal deaths.

In order to provide a more adequate basis for generalization from the Standard Records to the whole population, it was decided to reject varying proportions of these records, depending upon multiplicity (1 and 2 or more) birth weight (below 2,501 g and above 2,500 g) and outcome (late fetal death, early neonatal death, late neonatal death, survived for 1 month), with the object of obtaining an 'edited' set of Standard Records with a similar distribution of multiplicity, birth weight and outcome of delivery as the complete population of births (excluding those with unknown data). The proportions of records in each of the $2 \times 2 \times 4 = 16$ categories to be rejected in order to achieve this goal with the minimum loss of observations were calculated: the results varied from zero to 0.59. Each of the Standard Records was then assessed in turn, the category to which the individual record belonged was determined and a randomized procedure was followed by which a decision as to whether that particular record should be accepted or rejected was made. This decision was based upon the generation of a pseudo-random number sequence — standardized to the range (0, 1) — using a method of congruential multiplication, the record being accepted if the corresponding number in the sequence was less than or equal to the proportion of records to be retained appropriate to that category, and rejected otherwise. In this way, the 5,734 Standard Records were reduced to a total of 4,794, corresponding to the rejection of some 16.5% of the original Standard Records. The distribution of the three attributes amongst the edited Standard Records is shown below in table Ic. The proportions in each of the categories are similar to those in the whole population (table Ib), the small differences in the prevalences of certain of the less common classes reflecting random variations associated with the selection process.

The rejection procedure was successful in bringing the distribution of multiplicity, birth weight and outcome in the edited Standard Records into line with that in the whole population of births. The use of a randomized procedure for deciding which particular records should be rejected has secured this process against any possibility of bias. However, it is not in general possible to determine whether each item of information is present in the edited Standard Records in the same proportions as in the whole population of births. As a direct consequence of the procedures used to allocate births to the Standard Records, it is not feasible to ensure that district of residence (within the Municipality of Palermo) nor place of delivery appear in the appropriate proportions in the edited Standard Records. However, sex and maternal age are the two remaining items other than the selection variables which were recorded on all types of record and in each case the distribution in the edited Standard Records corresponds very closely to those in the complete population. Although there can be no conclusive proof that a similar result holds for any of the items whose distribution cannot be compared, these results, coupled with the good agreement of the birth weight distributions when expressed in detailed form (as opposed to the below 2,501-gram and above 2,500-gram groups), suggest that the editing process has achieved its main objectives. In the absence of evidence to the contrary, the edited Standard Records have been regarded as representative of the whole population in the statistical analysis.

Appendix 3

MEDICAL BIRTH RECORD

MOTHER

Code No Hospital	Department	Ward	(Place for citograph plate print giving national identity number, name, address, etc.)
Record No.	Referred by	Summary sent	

National identity No (year,month,day of birth reg. No)		Cause of admittance	

District insurance No	Parish code No	Child welfare clinic No	Spare box

Admission year month day	Marital status single ☐ married ☐ prev married ☐	Language (if not Swedish)

Discharge year month day	Alive to home ☐ another hosp ☐ another dept ☐ another addr ☐	Dead post mort ☐ no post mort ☐

Father's national identity No (year, month, day of birth, reg. No)   Address at discharge if different from above

PREVIOUS PREGNANCIES				PRESENT PREGNANCY			ANTENATAL CARE					BODY MEASURES	
Number	Still-births	Live-births	Deaths within 7 days	Date of last pregnancy year,month	LMP year month day	Gestational age in weeks	Information on gest.age were the date certain cer-tain ☐ uncer-tain ☐	Ante-natal clinic ☐	Priv. Dr ☐	None ☐	No of visits to dr to mid-wife	First visit in week No	Height cm	Weight before pregn. kg

COMPLICATION of present pregnancy

Diagnostic code StI x)	Diagnosis	☐ No complication

X) StI = Significant to infant

TYPE OF DELIVERY AND COMPLICATION TO IT   ☐ Puerperium uneventful

Diagnostic code StI	Diagnosis	ANALGESIA code (pain relief) oral ☐ parenta ☐

OBSTETRIC TREATMENT

Procedure Code StI	Procedure	ANESTHESIA code (at surgical operation)

INFANT

Infant record No (hospital identification No)

Date and time of birth year month day	time	Multiple birth order	No of infants	Single birth ☐	Sex M F ? ☐☐☐	Live birth ☐	Stillbirth dead before ☐ during labor	Weight of infant at birth	at discharge	Length at birth	at dis-charge	Head circumf. at birth	at dis-charge	Apgar score 1 min	5 min	min

NEONATAL COURSE (include cause of death of infant or stillbirth if appropriate)   Lowest weight

Diagnostic code	grade of severity	Diagnosis

NEONATAL TREATMENT

Code	Treatment

Discharge year month day	Alive to home ☐ pediat-ric ward ☐ another dept ☐ another addr. ☐	Date and time of death year month day	time	Post mort ☐	No post mort ☐	Number of in-patient days (total)	Number in neo-natal unit	in pediat ward	in another dept	Number of day in mother and baby room

Risk-factors	Type of follow-up at child welfare clinic ☐	early visit home ☐	date pediatr. ☐	Another date special service ☐	Feeding at discharge by breast-milk (ml) ☐ artificial feeding (ml)	Metabolic screening yes ☐ no ☐	BCG yes ☐ no ☐

Signature

Original: Record sheet for maternity or institution.
Copy 1: Medical notification of birth from maternity hospital to child welfare clinic.
Copy 2: Medical notification of birth from maternity hospital to antenatal clinic
Copy 3: Medical notification of birth from maternity hospital to the National Board of Health and Welfare (Data processing form)

Appendix 4

FÖRLOSSNINGSVÅRD 2 BARN Nr

JOURNAL

Födelsetid			Flerbörd född av nr | ant	Enkel börd	Kön g f ?	Lev född	Dödfött, dött före förl	under förl
år mån dag	klockan							

KROPPSMÅTT	Vikt, g	Längd, cm	Huvud-omf. cm	GRAVIDITETSLÄNGD		
				Graviditetsveckor	Uppgift om graviditetslängd	
vid födelsen						
vid utskrivn					säker	o-säker
lägsta vikt		Reserv				

FÖDELSE-ANMÄLAN	CFU	BVC / SoS	Med föd med till datum	sign

APGAR BEDÖMN	1 min	5 min	Poäng 0	1	2
Hjärtfrekv			ingen	< 100 oreg, långsam	> 100 god skriker
Andning			ingen	blek, cyanot	perif cyanos
Hudfärg			blek, cyanot	ned-satt	skär aktiva rörelser
Muskeltonus			slapp	grima-ser	nyser, hostar
Retbarhet			ingen reaktion		
Summa					

IAKTTAGELSER PÅ BARN UNDER 3.000 GRAM

Subcutant fettskikt	rikligt	sparsamt	saknas
Hudfärg ...	rosa	blek	mörkröd
Muskeltonus i extremiteter	kraftig i övre o nedre	god i nedre	nedsatt i övre o nedre
Bröstkörtel-storlek	> 6 mm	3–6 mm	< 3 mm
Fotsule-hudveck	rikligt hel fot	främre 2/3	främre 1/3

FÖDELSEVIKT och -LÄNGD
vid olika GRAVIDITETSTID
Medelvärden ± 2 SD
Pojkar: hel linje flickor: streckad linje

LÄNGD

Lång för tiden (778,15)

Kort för tiden (777,30)

Tung för tiden (778,11)

VIKT

Lätt för tiden (777,10)

Låg födelsevikt (777,20)

Underburen (777,00)   Fullgången   Överburen (778,10)

enl Engström, L.,Karlberg,P,Olsson,T-Selstam,U 1971 Copyright

DIAGNOSER (tillämpbart inringas)

Y 89, 09 Neonatalperioden u a

Andra diagnoser: Se ovan och baksidan

OMEDELBARA OCH ÖVRIGA ÅTGÄRDER / OBSERVATIONER						IDENTITETS-KONTROLL
	trachealtub			ja nej	Sign	på förlossnings-avd
Svalgtoalett Ventrikeltöm-ning	utan | med		Gom hel		Ögon-desinf 1 % lapis	
Trachealtoalett	behandling i min		Anus öp			
Mun-mot-mun-andning			K-vitamin (dos)			på vårdavd
Ej övertryck, luft			Andra åtgärder			
„ extra O₂						vid utskrivn
Övertryck, luft						
„ extra O₂						
Hjärtmassage (min)						
Anteckningar						

STATUS (avvikel-ser anges 0, 1, 2, 3)	dag/mån				Anteckningar
	klockan				
Undersökare					
Utseende					
Cyanos					
Icterus					
Spont rörelser					
Cor					
biljud					
Femoralis puls					
Respiration mönster					
Skalle font tension					
Rygg Övr skelett					
Reflex: Moro Grip-hand Grip-fot Sug					
Hypotonus Hypertonus					
Buk Navel Turgor					
Genitalia Höfter					
Svalg Vitalitet					

Missbildning (se baksidan)	Ja	Nej	Rapporterad till SoS		
Utskriven år mån dag	Levande till				
	hem-met	barn-klin	annan klin	annan	

Dött år mån dag	klockan	Obd	Ej obd	Vård-dagar totalt	därav på neonat avd	barn-klinik	annan klinik	Samvård mor-barn antal dagar

Rekommenderad hälsokontroll (0–3)	vid BVC	tidigt hembesök	barn spec	datum	annan spec	datum

Uppfödning vid utskrivning bröstmjölk, (ml)	ersättn prep, (ml)	Metabolscreen			BCG
		Ja	Nej	datum	
					Ja Nej

Övr anteckn på baksidan

SoS BS 1.05. Fastställd 24.3 1972

LIC MBF-6

Appendix 5

Anteckningar:

Appendix 6

MOTHER

MEDICAL BIRTH RECORD

Code No Hospital	Department	Ward	
503	401	14	
Record No. 858	Referred by		Summary sent

(Place for citograph plate print giving national identity number, name, address, etc.)

National identity No (year,month,day of birth reg. No)	Cause of admittance	
XXXXXX-XXXX	Onset of labour	

ABCDEFGH   XXXXXX-XXXX

District insurance No 3800	Parish code No 148019	Child welfare clinic No 32077	Spare box

XXXXXXXX

Admission year month day	Marital status	Language (if not Swedish)
76 02 12	☐ single ☐ married ☒ prev married	

XXXXX

Discharge year month day	Alive to	Dead no
76 02 17	☐ home ☐ another hosp ☐ another dept ☐ another addr	☐ post mort ☐ no post mort

Father's national identity No (year, month, day of birth, reg. No)	Address at discharge if different from above
XXXXXX-XXXX ABCDEFGHR	

PREVIOUS PREGNANCIES | PRESENT PREGNANCY | ANTENATAL CARE | BODY MEASURES

Number	Still-births	Live-births	Deaths within 7 days	Date of last pregnancy year,month	LMP year month day	Gestational age in weeks	Information on gest.age were the date certain cer- uncer-tain	Ante-natal clinic	Priv. Dr	None	No of visits to dr to mid-wife	First visit in week No	Height cm	Weight before pregn. kg
1	0	1	0	73 09	75 05 20	38	☒tain ☐tain	☒	☐	☐				

COMPLICATION of present pregnancy		☒ No complication
Diagnostic code StI x)	Diagnosis	
	X) StI = Significant to infant	

TYPE OF DELIVERY AND COMPLICATION TO IT	☐ Puerperium uneventful	ANALGESIA
Diagnostic code StI	Diagnosis	code (pain relief)
650.00	Partus normalis	oral ☐ parental ☐

OBSTETRIC TREATMENT		ANESTHESIA
Procedure Code StI	Procedure	code (at surgical operation)

INFANT

Infant record No
(hospital identification No)

Date and time of birth year month day time	Multiple birth birth / No of order infants	Single birth	Sex M F ?	Live birth dead	Stillbirth before during labor	Weight of infant at birth / at discharge	Length at birth / dis-charge	Head circumf. at birth / at dis-charge	Apgar score 1 min / 5 min / min
76 02 12 0259		☒	☒ ☐	☐	☐ ☐	2960 2930	48	33 34	9

Lowest weight

NEONATAL COURSE (include cause of death of infant or stillbirth if appropriate)	
Diagnostic code	grade of severity	Diagnosis
Y 89.99	Neonatal Course uneventful

NEONATAL TREATMENT	
Code	Treatment

Discharge year month day	Alive to home pediat-ric ward another dept another addr	Date and time of death year month day time	Post mort / No post mort	Number of in-patient days (total)	Number in neo-natal unit	in pediat ward	in another dept	Number of days in mother and baby room
76 02 17	☒ ☐ ☐ ☐		☐ ☐	5				5

Risk-factors	Type of follow-up at child welfare clinic early visit home ward	date pediatr.	Another date special service	Feeding at discharge by breast-milk (ml) / artificial feeding (ml)	Metabolic screening yes no	BCG yes no
☒	☒ ☐ ☐		☐	☒ ☐	☒ ☐	☐ ☒

Signature	KLMNOPQRST

Original: Record sheet for maternity or institution.
Copy 1: Medical notification of birth from maternity hospital to child welfare clinic.
Copy 2: Medical notification of birth from maternity hospital to antenatal clinic
Copy 3: Medical notification of birth from maternity hospital to the National Board of Health and Welfare (Data processing form)

Appendix 7

MOTHER			
Code No Hospital **360**	Department **451**	Ward **14**	(Place for citograph plate print giving national identity number, name, address, etc.) ABCDEFGHR XXXXXX-XXXX XXXXXXXXX XXXXX
Record No. **453**	Referred by		
National identity No (year,month,day of birth reg. No) **XXXXXX-XXXX**	Cause of admittance **Onset of labor**		
District insurance No **3800**	Parish code No **148005**	Child welfare clinic No **3207**	Spare box
Admission year month day **75 12 05**	Marital status ☐single ☒married ☐prev married		Language (if not Swedish)
Discharge year month day **75 12 05**	Alive to ☒home ☐hosp ☐dept ☐addr another another another		Dead no post post ☐mort ☐mort
Father's national identity No (year, month, day of birth, reg. No) **XXXXXX-XXXX ABCDE**			Address at discharge if different from above

PREVIOUS PREGNANCIES

Number	Still-births	Live-births	Deaths within 7 days	Date of last pregnancy year,month
0	0	0	0	–

PRESENT PREGNANCY

LMP year month day	Gestational age in weeks	Information on gest.age were the date certain
75 02 10	41	cer-tain ☒ uncer-tain ☐

ANTENATAL CARE

Ante-natal clinic	Priv. Dr	None	No of visits to dr/to mid-wife	First visit in week No
☐	☐	☐		

☒ No complication

BODY MEASURES

Height cm	Weight before pregn. kg

COMPLICATION of present pregnancy

Diagnostic code StI x)	Diagnosis

X) StI = Significant to infant

TYPE OF DELIVERY AND COMPLICATION TO IT   ☐ Puerperium uneventful

Diagnostic code StI	Diagnosis
661.78-3	Partus complicatus ex asphyxia fetus intrauterina immeco
672.99	Febris puerperalis incertae cause

ANALGESIA code (pain relief)   oral ☐   parental ☒

OBSTETRIC TREATMENT

Procedure Code StI	Procedure
7810	Cesarian section (abominal section of lower uterine segment)
9320	Injection anti-D

ANESTHESIA code (at surgical operation)

Infant record No (hospital identification No) **6535**

INFANT			
Date and time of birth year month day / time **75 11 25 / 0900**	Multiple birth / birth order / No of infants ☒	Single birth	Sex M F ? ☒☐☐

Live birth	Stillbirth dead before / during labor	Weight of infant at birth / at discharge	Length at birth / at discharge	Head circumf. at birth / at discharge	Apgar score 1 min / 5 min / min
☐	☐ ☐	3360	51	35	6

Lowest weight **3280**

NEONATAL COURSE (include cause of death of infant or stillbirth if appropriate)

Diagnostic code	grade of severity	Diagnosis		
776.30-2		Asphyxia intrauterina	778.93-2	Hyperbilirubinemia
777.60		Dysmaturitas	746.97-1	VOC? (VSD?)
776.00-3		Syndroma aspirationes		

NEONATAL TREATMENT

Code	Treatment
9380	Use of incubator
9370	Oxygentheraphy
9340	Umbilical artery cathode

Discharge year month day **75 12 22**	Alive to ☒home ☐pediatric ward ☐another dept ☐another addr.	Date and time of death year month day / time	Post mort ☐ / No post mort ☐	Number of in-patient days (total) **27**	Number in neo-natal unit	in pedia ward	in another dept **27**	Number of days in mother and baby room

Risk-factors	Type of follow-up at child welfare clinic ☒ / early visit home ☐ / date pediatr. ☒	Another date special service ☐	Feeding at discharge by breast-milk (ml) / artificial feeding (ml) ☐	Metabolic screening yes no ☐ ☒	BCG yes no ☒ ☐

Signature **KLMNOPQRS**